T0263939

Advancements in Clinical Laryngology

Editors

JONATHAN M. BOCK
CHANDRA M. IVEY
KAREN B. ZUR

OTOLARYNGOLOGIC CLINICS OF NORTH AMERICA

www.oto.theclinics.com

Consulting Editor
SUJANA S. CHANDRASEKHAR

August 2019 • Volume 52 • Number 4

ELSEVIER

1600 John F. Kennedy Boulevard • Suite 1800 • Philadelphia, Pennsylvania, 19103-2899

http://www.oto.theclinics.com

OTOLARYNGOLOGIC CLINICS OF NORTH AMERICA Volume 52, Number 4
August 2019 ISSN 0030-6665, ISBN-13: 978-0-323-68240-4

Editor: Jessica McCool
Developmental Editor: Laura Kavanaugh

© **2019 Elsevier Inc. All rights reserved.**

This periodical and the individual contributions contained in it are protected under copyright by Elsevier, and the following terms and conditions apply to their use:

Photocopying

Single photocopies of single articles may be made for personal use as allowed by national copyright laws. Permission of the Publisher and payment of a fee is required for all other photocopying, including multiple or systematic copying, copying for advertising or promotional purposes, resale, and all forms of document delivery. Special rates are available for educational institutions that wish to make photocopies for non-profit educational classroom use. For information on how to seek permission visit www.elsevier.com/permissions or call: (+44) 1865 843830 (UK)/(+1) 215 239 3804 (USA).

Derivative Works

Subscribers may reproduce tables of contents or prepare lists of articles including abstracts for internal circulation within their institutions. Permission of the Publisher is required for resale or distribution outside the institution. Permission of the Publisher is required for all other derivative works, including compilations and translations (please consult www.elsevier.com/permissions).

Electronic Storage or Usage

Permission of the Publisher is required to store or use electronically any material contained in this periodical, including any article or part of an article (please consult www.elsevier.com/permissions). Except as outlined above, no part of this publication may be reproduced, stored in a retrieval system or transmitted in any form or by any means, electronic, mechanical, photocopying, recording or otherwise, without prior written permission of the Publisher.

Notice

No responsibility is assumed by the Publisher for any injury and/or damage to persons or property as a matter of products liability, negligence or otherwise, or from any use or operation of any methods, products, instructions or ideas contained in the material herein. Because of rapid advances in the medical sciences, in particular, independent verification of diagnoses and drug dosages should be made.

Although all advertising material is expected to conform to ethical (medical) standards, inclusion in this publication does not constitute a guarantee or endorsement of the quality or value of such product or of the claims made of it by its manufacturer.

Otolaryngologic Clinics of North America (ISSN 0030-6665) is published bimonthly by Elsevier, Inc., 360 Park Avenue South, New York, NY 10010-1710. Months of issue are February, April, June, August, October, and December. Business and Editorial Offices: 1600 John F. Kennedy Blvd., Suite 1800, Philadelphia, PA 19103-2899. Customer Service Office: 6277 Sea Harbor Drive, Orlando, FL 32887-4800. Periodicals postage paid at New York, NY and additional mailing offices. Subscription prices are $412.00 per year (US individuals), $889.00 per year (US institutions), $100.00 per year (US student/resident), $548.00 per year (Canadian individuals), $1127.00 per year (Canadian institutions), $564.00 per year (international individuals), $1127.00 per year (international institutions), $270.00 per year (international & Canadian student/resident). Foreign air speed delivery is included in all *Clinics'* subscription prices. All prices are subject to change without notice. **POSTMASTER:** Send address changes to *Otolaryngologic Clinics of North America*, Elsevier Health Sciences Division, Subscription Customer Service, 3251 Riverport Lane, Maryland Heights, MO 63043. **Telephone: 1-800-654-2452 (U.S. and Canada); 314-447-8871 (outside U.S. and Canada). Fax: 314-447-8029. E-mail: journalscustomerservice-usa@elsevier.com (for print support); journalsonlinesupport-usa@elsevier.com (for online support).**

Reprints. For copies of 100 or more of articles in this publication, please contact the Commercial Reprints Department, Elsevier Inc., 360 Park Avenue South, New York, NY 10010-1710. Tel.: 212-633-3874; Fax: 212-633-3820; E-mail: reprints@elsevier.com.

Otolaryngologic Clinics of North America is also published in Spanish by McGraw-Hill Interamericana Editores S.A., P.O. Box 5-237, 06500 Mexico D.F., Mexico.

Otolaryngologic Clinics of North America is covered in *MEDLINE/PubMed (Index Medicus), Current Contents/Clinical Medicine, Excerpta Medica, BIOSIS, Science Citation Index,* and *ISI/BIOMED.*

Contributors

CONSULTING EDITOR

SUJANA S. CHANDRASEKHAR, MD, FACS, FAAOHNS
Past President, American Academy of Otolaryngology–Head and Neck Surgery, Partner,
ENT & Allergy Associates, LLP, Clinical Professor, Department of Otolaryngology–Head
and Neck Surgery, Zucker School of Medicine at Hofstra-Northwell, Hempstead, New
York, USA; Clinical Associate Professor, Department of Otolaryngology–Head and Neck
Surgery, Icahn School of Medicine at Mount Sinai, New York, New York, USA

EDITORS

JONATHAN M. BOCK, MD, FACS
Associate Professor, Division of Laryngology and Professional Voice, Department of
Otolaryngology–Head and Neck Surgery and Communication Sciences, Medical College
of Wisconsin, Milwaukee, Wisconsin, USA

CHANDRA M. IVEY, MD, FACS
Assistant Clinical Professor, Department of Otolaryngology–Head and Neck Surgery,
Icahn School of Medicine, Mount Sinai Hospital, New York, New York, USA

KAREN B. ZUR, MD
Director, Pediatric Voice Program, Children's Hospital of Philadelphia, Associate
Professor, Otolaryngology–Head AND Neck Surgery, Perelman School of Medicine,
University of Pennsylvania, Philadelphia, Pennsylvania, USA

AUTHORS

S. AHMED ALI, MD
Department of Otolaryngology–Head and Neck Surgery, Michigan Medicine, Ann Arbor,
Michigan, USA

ANDREW E. BLUHER, MD
Resident Physician, Department of Otolaryngology–Head and Neck Surgery,
Eastern Virginia Medical School, Sentara Norfolk General Hospital, Norfolk, Virginia,
USA

JONATHAN M. BOCK, MD, FACS
Associate Professor, Division of Laryngology and Professional Voice, Department of
Otolaryngology–Head and Neck Surgery and Communication Sciences, Medical College
of Wisconsin, Milwaukee, Wisconsin, USA

PAUL C. BRYSON, MD
Head, Section of Laryngology, Director, Cleveland Clinic Voice Center, Associate
Professor of Otolaryngology–Head and Neck Surgery, Cleveland Clinic Lerner College of
Medicine, Case Western Reserve University, Cleveland, Ohio, USA

THOMAS L. CARROLL, MD
Director, Brigham and Women's Voice Program, Brigham and Women's Hospital, Assistant Professor, Department of Otolaryngology–Head and Neck Surgery, Harvard Medical School, Boston, Massachusetts, USA

JULIANA CODINO, MS, CCC-SLP
Lakeshore Professional Voice Center, Lakeshore Ear, Nose & Throat Center, St Clair Shores, Michigan, USA; University of Buenos Aires, Buenos Aires, Argentina

MARK S. COUREY, MD
Professor, Otolaryngology–Head and Neck Surgery, Division Chief, Laryngology, Vice Chair of Quality, Department of Otolaryngology–Head and Neck Surgery, Icahn School of Medicine at Mount Sinai, New York, New York, USA

SETH H. DAILEY, MD
Division of Otolaryngology–Head and Neck Surgery, Department of Surgery, University of Wisconsin Hospital and Clinics, Madison, Wisconsin, USA

CRAIG S. DERKAY, MD, FACS, FAAP
Professor and Vice Chairman, Department of Otolaryngology–Head and Neck Surgery, Director, Pediatric Otolaryngology, Eastern Virginia Medical School, Children's Hospital of the King's Daughters, Norfolk, Virginia, USA

ERIN NICOLE DONAHUE, BM, MA, CCC-SLP
Voice Pathologist and Singing Voice Specialist, Clinical Organization and Outreach Lead, The Blaine Block Institute for Voice Analysis and Rehabilitation, Dayton, Ohio, USA; The Professional Voice Center of Greater Cincinnati, Cincinnati, Ohio, USA

DAVID O. FRANCIS, MD, MS
Associate Professor of Surgery, Division of Otolaryngology–Head and Neck Surgery, Wisconsin Surgical Outcomes Research Program, Department of Surgery, University of Wisconsin–Madison, Madison, Wisconsin, USA

M. ELISE GRAHAM, MD, FRCSC
Assistant Professor, Department of Otolaryngology–Head and Neck Surgery, Children's Hospital at London Health Sciences Centre, Schulich School of Medicine and Dentistry, Western University, London, Ontario, Canada

MINGYANG L. GRAY, MD, MPH
Resident Physician, Department of Otolaryngology–Head and Neck Surgery, Icahn School of Medicine at Mount Sinai, New York, New York, USA

ELIZABETH GUARDIANI, MD
Assistant Professor of Otorhinolaryngology–Head and Neck Surgery, University of Maryland School of Medicine, Baltimore, Maryland, USA

NORMAN D. HOGIKYAN, MD, FACS
Professor, Department of Otolaryngology–Head and Neck Surgery, Michigan Medicine, Ann Arbor, Michigan, USA

TIFFINY A. HRON, MD
Instructor, Harvard Medical School, Adjunct Clinical Instructor, Tufts University School of Medicine, Massachusetts General Hospital, Center for Laryngeal Surgery and Voice Rehabilitation, Boston, Massachusetts, USA

INNA HUSAIN, MD
Rush University Medical Center, Chicago, Illinois, USA

CHANDRA M. IVEY, MD, FACS
Assistant Clinical Professor, Department of Otolaryngology–Head and Neck Surgery, Icahn School of Medicine, Mount Sinai Hospital, New York, New York, USA

KATHERINE R. KAVANAGH, MD
Director of Research, Pediatric Otolaryngology, Connecticut Children's Medical Center, Hartford, Connecticut, USA; Associate Professor, Department of Otolaryngology–Head and Neck Surgery, University of Connecticut School of Medicine, Farmington, Connecticut, USA

KRISTEN L. KRAIMER, BS
Rush Medical College, Chicago, Illinois, USA

WENDY DELEO LEBORGNE, BFA, MA, PhD, CCC-SLP
Clinical Director, Voice Pathologist and Singing Voice Specialist, The Blaine Block Institute for Voice Analysis and Rehabilitation, Dayton, Ohio, USA; The Professional Voice Center of Greater Cincinnati, University of Cincinnati, Adjunct Associate Professor, CCM/TAPAA, Musical Theater, Cincinnati, Ohio, USA

NICOLE MURRAY, MD
Director, Center for Airway, Voice, and Swallowing Disorders, Connecticut Children's Medical Center, Hartford, Connecticut, USA; Associate Professor, Department of Otolaryngology–Head and Neck Surgery, University of Connecticut Medical School, Farmington, Connecticut, USA

DEBBIE R. PAN, BA
Department of Otolaryngology, University of Miami Miller School of Medicine, Miami, Florida, USA

SARANYA REGHUNATHAN, MD
Laryngology Fellow, Cleveland Clinic, Cleveland, Ohio, USA

DAVID E. ROSOW, MD, FACS
Director, Division of Laryngology and Voice, Associate Professor, Department of Otolaryngology, University of Miami Miller School of Medicine, Miami, Florida, USA

ADAM D. RUBIN, MD
Lakeshore Professional Voice Center, Lakeshore Ear, Nose & Throat Center, St Clair Shores, Michigan, USA; Oakland University William Beaumont School of Medicine, Rochester, Michigan, USA; Michigan State University College of Osteopathic Medicine, University of Michigan, Michigan, USA

JOSHUA D. SMITH, BA
Department of Otolaryngology–Head and Neck Surgery, Michigan Medicine, Ann Arbor, Michigan, USA

LIBBY J. SMITH, DO
Associate Professor of Otolaryngology, Department of Otolaryngology–Head and Neck Surgery, University of Pittsburgh, Eye & Ear Institute, Pittsburgh, Pennsylvania, USA

MARSHALL E. SMITH, MD, FACS
Professor, Division of Otolaryngology–Head and Neck Surgery, University of Utah School of Medicine, Salt Lake City, Utah, USA

GRACE SNOW, MD
Resident, Otorhinolaryngology Head and Neck Surgery, University of Maryland School of Medicine, Baltimore, Maryland, USA

RESHA S. SONI, MD
Division of Otolaryngology–Head and Neck Surgery, Department of Surgery, University of Wisconsin Hospitals and Clinics, Madison, Wisconsin, USA

MELIN TAN-GELLER, MD
Associate Professor, Department of Otolaryngology, Albert Einstein College of Medicine, Bronx, New York, USA

RALUCA TAVALUC, MD
Department of Head and Neck Surgery, University of California, Los Angeles, Los Angeles, California, USA

SUNIL P. VERMA, MD
Associate Professor, Department of Otolaryngology–Head and Neck Surgery, University of California, Irvine, Orange, California, USA

ALISA ZHUKHOVITSKAYA, MD
Resident Physician, Department of Otolaryngology–Head and Neck Surgery, University of California, Irvine, Orange, California, USA

Contents

This article provides a concise review of contemporary options for evaluating voice disorders. Focus is given to patient history and patient-derived voice handicap and quality of life assessments, clinician-derived perceptual analysis of voice, and finally flexible and rigid, high-definition laryngoscopy with videostroboscopy to fully evaluate laryngeal function and biomechanics.

The Hoarseness Guideline Update provides an evidence-based approach to a patient who presents to the clinic with hoarseness. The guidelines cover management decisions in acute and chronic dysphonia for patients of all ages before and after laryngeal examination. The present review discusses the process used to develop these guidelines, including limitations of the process and each key action statement.

Chronic laryngitis is an inflammatory process of at least 3 weeks duration and affects phonation, breathing, and swallowing. This article describes the infectious, inflammatory, and autoimmune causes of chronic laryngitis. Symptoms of chronic laryngitis are nonspecific and may range from mild to airway compromise requiring emergent tracheostomy.

Presbyphonia is defined as aging of the voice, and its growing attention as a medical concern parallels the continuing increase of the geriatric population worldwide. It results from physiologic changes to several laryngeal structures, including the musculature, surrounding cartilage, and lamina propria of the vocal folds. Characterized by glottic insufficiency, dysphonia in the elderly typically presents as a deterioration of voice quality, altered pitch and fundamental frequency, vocal fatigue, and strain. Fortunately,

lesions of the larynx in pediatrics are vocal nodules, vocal fold polyps, cysts, granulomas, ectasias, sulcus vocalis, and vascular lesions, including hemangioma and postcricoid cushion. Treatment of benign vocal lesions should be tailored to the individual patient and the perceived impact.

Recurrent respiratory papillomatosis (RRP) remains a challenging disease afflicting children and adults, resulting in an estimated $120 million per year in United States healthcare–related costs, with annual costs per patient approaching $60,000. Although the prevalence of RRP has declined, RRP remains the most common benign laryngeal neoplasm in children. RRP is unique in its high rate of multisite recurrence, its high burden on patient quality of life, and its high associated healthcare costs. This article summarizes current understanding of the natural history and quality of life burden of RRP, and basic science advancements in prevention and treatment.

Unilateral vocal fold paralysis (UVFP) in children may cause dysfunction in voice, swallowing, and breathing, thus influencing all components of laryngeal function. UVFP in children is usually the result of iatrogenic injury. The approach to patients with suspected UVFP should involve a detailed patient history, a focused physical examination with flexible nasopharyngoscopy, and relevant imaging if the cause of UVFP is uncertain. Management aims to strengthen voice, decrease aspiration, and improve quality of life. Laryngeal reinnervation is becoming more common, potentially offering permanent improvement in vocal and swallowing function through increasing bulk and tone to the paralyzed vocal fold.

Medications can have innumerable direct and indirect effects on laryngeal hydration, vocal fold mucosal integrity, laryngeal muscle function, and laryngeal sensation. Effects, therefore, can be subtle and slowly progressive over time. This article delineates the general classes of medications that are known to cause alterations of vocal function, highlights medical history symptoms that may help raise suspicion for medication-related vocal changes, and presents recommendations for approaches to treatment of these issues.

Laryngeal mucosal precursor lesions represent a challenging clinical entity. Updated classification systems allow for grade-based categorization. Multiple management options exist, with treatment decisions made jointly by physician and patient and focused on both appropriate lesion treatment and preservation of laryngeal structure and function. Traditional methods include cold steel and CO_2 laser excision, with newer modalities using angiolytic lasers for lesion ablation. Both operating room–based and office-based treatment options exist, and there are advantages and disadvantages to each approach. Research is ongoing to advance the understanding of lesion biology, and to optimize prevention and treatment.

Voice is a complex marker for gender and pivotal to the gender reassignment process. The goal of the transgender patient is to achieve a voice and communication style that is congruent with their gender identity. Voice and speech therapy are fundamental for successful transition. Phonosurgery, to adjust pitch, can be an important adjunct to relieve the patient from active pitch elevation of voice to free them to focus on the other adjustments needed and learned through behavioral training with speech and voice therapy. The authors review current management options for transgender patients with difficulties in voice and communication style.

Dysphonia is often blamed on laryngopharyngeal reflux (LPR) in the face of a normal flexible laryngoscopic examination. LPR remains primarily (and unfortunately) a diagnosis of exclusion rather than inclusion in the face of vague throat complaints and laryngeal signs attributed to reflux. LPR remains misdiagnosed and overdiagnosed as the cause of many identical, vague throat symptoms and laryngeal complaints. Despite LPR being commonly implicated as the cause of a myriad of nonspecific pharyngeal symptoms, LPR as a physiologic process is common. Whether or not it is a contributor to a patient's symptoms, especially dysphonia, is the focus of this article.

Sulcus vocalis, defined as a type of groove along the free edge of the vocal fold, disrupts the normal, pliable vocal fold cover, causing alterations in the intrinsic mucosal wave. The primary symptom is breathy, effortful dysphonia. Diagnosis may be challenging, and this classically has led to difficulties with identification and management. Treatment options, although often promising, have been notoriously unreliable. Current understanding, considerations for management, and future treatment options are explored.

 Video content accompanies this article at http://www.oto.theclinics.com.

Benign laryngeal lesions are often the result of phonotraumatic forces on the vocal folds and thus classically are treated with a combination of voice therapy and phonomicrosurgical techniques to minimize inadvertent additional trauma. Newer management strategies expand on these techniques with the use of the pKTP laser as well as intralesional injections, both in the operating room and in the awake outpatient setting.

Movement Disorders and Voice

Grace Snow and Elizabeth Guardiani

The primary movement disorders affecting the voice are laryngeal dystonia (including spasmodic dysphonia), essential voice tremor, and Parkinson disease. Diagnosis of these conditions is clinical and based on a detailed history, voice evaluation, and physical and laryngoscopic examination. Laryngeal dystonia and essential voice tremor are hyperfunctional disorders and are treated most commonly with botulinum toxin injections. Parkinson disease is a hypofunctional disorder that may affect the voice and most commonly is treated with Lee Silverman Voice Treatment.

The Art of Caring for the Professional Singer

Adam D. Rubin and Juliana Codino

Training in care of the voice for the general otolaryngologist has improved with the presence of more fellowship-trained laryngologists within academic training programs. However, preparation for caring for the professional singer goes beyond the basic understanding of voice evaluation, laryngeal imaging, and microlaryngeal surgery. The otolaryngologist must have a deeper understanding of the demands, vocabulary, psyche, and economics of the professional singer to provide optimal care. The ramification of recommendations made or procedures undertaken by the otolaryngologist can have serious consequences in a singer's career. This article introduces the otolaryngologist to the specifics of caring for professional singers.

OTOLARYNGOLOGIC CLINICS
OF NORTH AMERICA

FORTHCOMING ISSUES

October 2019
Updates in Pediatric Otolaryngology
Samantha Anne and Julina Ongkasuwan,
Editors

December 2019
Anesthesia for Otolaryngology
Adam I. Levine, Samuel DeMaria Jr, and
Satish Govindaraj, *Editors*

February 2020
**Cranial Nerve Stimulation in
Otolaryngology**
James G. Naples and Michael J.
Ruckenstein, *Editors*

RECENT ISSUES

June 2019
Office-Based Surgery in Otolaryngology
Melissa A. Pynnonen and
Cecelia E. Schmalbach, *Editors*

April 2019
Implantable Auditory Devices
Darius Kohan and
Sujana S. Chandrasekhar, *Editors*

February 2019
Patient Safety and Quality Improvement
Rahul K. Shah, *Editor*

SERIES OF RELATED INTEREST

Facial Plastic Surgery Clinics
Available at: https://www.facialplastic.theclinics.com/

THE CLINICS ARE AVAILABLE ONLINE!
Access your subscription at:
www.theclinics.com

Foreword

Improving Quality of Communication: Caring for All Voices

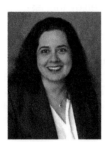

Sujana S. Chandrasekhar, MD, FACS, FAAOHNS
Consulting Editor

Of all creatures, humans use their voices most robustly. Communication can occur in many ways, but vocal communication is most refined in humans. We learn language starting in infancy, when we begin mimicking sounds and inflections, and then go on to make words and sentences. It is said that there is no more beautiful and complicated vocalization in nature than the human song. Our larynx, initially designed for airway protection, affords us the ability to express ourselves with voice, whispered, spoken, shouted, and sung. A certain combination of sound qualities allows one to identify their parent's voice or a favorite speaker or singer's voice amidst a babble of other sounds. The tone, pitch, quality of articulation, and inflection of our voices can make a critical difference in the way we are perceived and treated. When used effectively, our voice can work in our favor and enhance our personal and professional relationships.

Like many things, we don't know how much we value our voice until it changes or disappears. The care and feeding of the human larynx is to what this issue of *Otolaryngologic Clinics of North America* is dedicated. I commend Drs Bock, Ivey, and Zur on compiling a comprehensive resource that covers all of the important topics and pairs them with outstanding authors, who are thought leaders in the field.

Voice and larynx issues can occur at all ages, from infancy through geriatrics. Assessment of voice and laryngeal anatomy and physiology in a systematic manner allows for appropriate, targeted care. There are evidence-based guidelines on hoarseness based on systematic data review that are discussed here. Management of relatively common findings, such as Reinke edema, gastroesophageal reflux disease, chronic laryngitis, benign and premalignant lesions, and sulcus vocalis, is covered in a way that gives the reader the up-to-date information that is needed for office-based voice care. Special populations, such as children, the elderly, people with generalized

Otolaryngol Clin N Am 52 (2019) xiii–xiv
https://doi.org/10.1016/j.otc.2019.05.001
0030-6665/19/© 2019 Published by Elsevier Inc.

movement disorders, transgender individuals, and singers, all merit knowledgeable care, and the articles devoted to them provide succinct and comprehensive advice on assessment and management for their voice and larynx concerns. Although otolaryngologists work closely with speech therapists, they may not be thoroughly cognizant of how they assess and treat the patients. The article covering this is an excellent piece of education.

After reading through this issue of *Otolaryngologic Clinics of North America*, it is clear that there have been several advancements in all aspects of clinical laryngology. I again congratulate the Guest Editors, Drs Bock, Ivey, and Zur, and all of the authors, on this excellent, easily readable reference. I hope you enjoy this issue as much as I did. Look out for the podcast on the issue later at www.oto.theclinics.com. It is hoped our voices will all sound nicely clear and resonant to your ears!

Sujana S. Chandrasekhar, MD, FACS, FAAOHNS
Past President, American Academy of Otolaryngology-Head and Neck Surgery
Partner, ENT & Allergy Associates, LLP
Department of Otolaryngology–Head and Neck Surgery
Zucker School of Medicine at Hofstra-Northwell
Hempstead, NY, USA

Department of Otolaryngology–Head and Neck Surgery
Icahn School of Medicine at Mount Sinai
New York, NY, USA

ENT & Allergy Associates, LLP
18 East 48th Street, 2nd Floor
New York, NY 10017, USA

E-mail address:
ssc@nyotology.com

Preface

Advancements in Clinical Laryngology

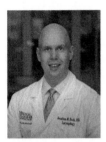 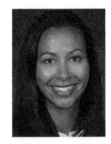 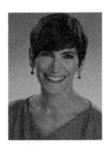

Jonathan M. Bock, MD, FACS   Chandra M. Ivey, MD, FACS   Karen B. Zur, MD

Editors

As with many medical specialties, Otolaryngology has been moving toward subspecialization. Through the hard work of interested innovators in both general otolaryngology and head and neck surgical specialties, Laryngology has developed into a highly specialized and scientific field. The last decade has seen a steep rise in specialists getting trained in voice health. Clinical and bench research on subjects of vocal tract physiology, voice production and pathology, and techniques for addressing these problems is being published in high-level journals. These are providing justification for Laryngology necessitating additional education as a fellowship for proficiency.

This issue of *Otolaryngology Clinics of North America* seeks to disseminate clinical advancements in laryngology to all Otolaryngologists who see patients with voice complaints and who have an interest in managing these problems within their practice. We have included articles that summarize and update fundamental elements of clinical laryngology care and review current knowledge and thoughts on these topics. These include components of voice evaluation, identification and management of chronic laryngitis, voice therapy for primary treatment of vocal fold pathology, vocal fold hyperkeratosis and dysplasia, and updated medical and surgical treatment for common benign laryngeal lesions. The most current clinical practice guideline on management of hoarseness has been included in a concise, understandable way. Newer topics focus on presbyphonia and minimal glottic insufficiency, Reinke's edema, transgender voice, vocal fold paresis, recurrent respiratory papillomatosis, sulcus vocalis, and voice-specific pediatric articles (diagnosis and treatment of benign pediatric lesions and unilateral vocal fold immobility in children). As a reminder that laryngologic issues can be impacted by other medical conditions, we have included articles on medications, gastroesophageal reflux, and movement disorders. We also discuss the art of caring for the professional singer.

Otolaryngol Clin N Am 52 (2019) xv–xvi
https://doi.org/10.1016/j.otc.2019.04.002
0030-6665/19/© 2019 Published by Elsevier Inc.

Due to the great volume and value of information on the above-mentioned voice-related topics, this issue does not cover swallowing disorders and their management, as an entire publication will be necessary to cover this facet of Laryngology. We have thoroughly enjoyed the privilege of editing this issue and hope this information is meaningful and useful to clinical practice of our specialty.

Jonathan M. Bock, MD, FACS
Division of Laryngology & Professional Voice
Department of Otolaryngology and Communication Sciences
Medical College of Wisconsin
8701 Watertown Plank Road
Milwaukee, WI 53226, USA

Chandra M. Ivey, MD, FACS
Department of Otolaryngology
Head and Neck Surgery
Icahn School of Medicine
Mount Sinai Hospital
210 East 86th Street, 9th Floor
New York, NY 10028, USA

Karen B. Zur, MD
Pediatric Voice Program
Children's Hospital of Philadelphia
Otolaryngology: Head & Neck Surgery
Perelman School of Medicine
University of Pennsylvania
3401 Civic Center Boulevard
1 Wood Ent
Philadelphia, PA 19104, USA

E-mail addresses:
jbock@mcw.edu (J.M. Bock)
civey@entandallergy.com (C.M. Ivey)
zur@email.chop.edu (K.B. Zur)

Components of Voice Evaluation

Saranya Reghunathan, MD[a], Paul C. Bryson, MD[b],*

KEYWORDS

- Voice • Laryngoscopy • Stroboscopy • Voice evaluation • VHI • GRBAS • CAPE-V

KEY POINTS

- There are several components to evaluating voice complaints: patient history, perceptual voice evaluation, physical examination, and videostroboscopic evaluation.
- Voice evaluation requires assessment of the respiratory system, the larynx, and the resonance capabilities of the upper airway.
- Clinicians should develop a system that works for their practice to include patient-derived surveys that are concise, informative, and repeatable; perceptual analysis of voice that is easy to obtain before and after treatment; and finally, high image quality laryngoscopy equipment with stroboscopy that can be recorded, reviewed, and archived.

INTRODUCTION

Voice evaluation requires assessment of the respiratory system, the larynx, and the resonance capabilities of the upper airway. Normal phonation requires adequate breath support, approximation of the vocal folds, vocal fold pliability, and control of vocal fold length and tension.[1]

The patient's description of their voice changes as well as the perceived impact on daily function are critical for the diagnosis and treatment of voice disorders. This article focuses primarily on the speaking voice, with attention paid elsewhere to singing and performance voice.

HISTORY

Patients often complain of "hoarseness," which essentially corresponds to their perception of altered voice quality. Hoarseness can correspond to both a symptom and a sign of dysfunction anywhere in the phonatory apparatus. The first element of

Disclosure Statement: The authors have nothing to disclose.
[a] Cleveland Clinic, 9500 Euclid Avenue, A-71, Cleveland, OH 44195, USA; [b] Section of Laryngology, Cleveland Clinic Voice Center, 9500 Euclid Avenue, A-71, Cleveland, OH 44195, USA
* Corresponding author.
E-mail address: brysonp@ccf.org

voice evaluation is the interpretation of the patient's description and perception of the altered voice and the important personal and subjective considerations that influence the voice complaint.

The history should include the following components:

- Description of voice problem, including onset and variability of symptoms
  - Altered voice quality
  - Phonatory fatigue
  - Insufficient loudness
  - Restricted pitch range
  - Increased phonatory effort
  - Breathlessness or conversational dyspnea
  - Impaired singing quality or ability
- Past voice disorders and any treatments
- Past surgical history
- Past medical history and current medical status, chronic medical conditions
- Medications
- Other environmental factors (home and occupational)
- Voice habits and hygiene[2] (daily vocal load)

The purpose of this comprehensive assessment is to identify underlying difficulties or abnormalities in speech production. Oftentimes, other comorbid health conditions and medications can affect the voice and must be assessed. It is of special importance to understand the patient's limitations in vocal activity and participation, both personal and professional; this is best described as the patient's self-assessment. The patient may describe this as a functional limitation in communication or interpersonal interaction. A critical part of the history includes understanding which component of voice the patient finds most troublesome. This is sometimes different than what the clinician perceives as the most obvious abnormality to the voice. Patient observations of voice problems tend to be individual; it is important to understand the environmental and personal factors the patient identifies as barriers to successful communication. It is also important to note that some individuals have expectations of their voices that are not absolute occupational needs but still may be reported as limiting, both professionally and socially. Understanding the patient's perspective on how their voice abnormality impairs quality of life will give the otolaryngologist a sense of potential treatment options that will be accepted.

VOICE-SPECIFIC PATIENT-REPORTED QUESTIONNAIRES

Several patient surveys/questionnaires have been created and validated to provide clinicians insight to a patient's initial disability. Among them, the Voice Handicap Index-10 (VHI-10)[3] and the Voice-Related Quality of Life (VRQoL)[4] are the most widely used. Such inventories help understand patient motivation, so the physician can make appropriate treatment recommendations. The VHI-10, for example, delivers a multifaceted assessment, as it gives information on the functional, emotional, and physical attributes of a patient's voice disorder. Another survey, The Glottal Function Index (GFI), is a validated 4-item self-administered survey used to evaluate glottal insufficiency.[5] The GFI has been used as an alternative to the VHI due to its brevity and ease in use.[5] Applied both before and after treatment, self-assessments can be an important means for measuring outcomes; these can allow for comparison of interventions, techniques, and studies.

PERCEPTUAL EVALUATION OF VOICE

The auditory perceptual assessment of voice can be both formal and informal. The informal component occurs during the initial history. It involves engaging the patient in spontaneous conversation while obtaining relevant information. Voice quality, pitch range, resonance (normal, hypo- or hypernasal), loudness, prosody, and articulation can be generally assessed.[6]

In addition, it is critical to take note of any diplophonia, aphonia, tremor, vocal fry, falsetto, and wet sounding voice. Diplophonia is characterized by the perception of 2 simultaneous pitches in the voice. It can be seen in a variety of settings such as mass lesions, vocal fold paresis or paralysis, or other causes of glottic insufficiency. Vocal fry is described as a pharyngeally focused voice and can be seen in younger adults attempting to sound more mature or authoritative.

The formal perceptual assessment typically involves the use of a protocol to systematically describe and quantify various features of the voice. Although there are many schemes that have been described, 2 main protocols are commonly used. The first, GRBAS scale, is examiner based and is the gold standard in perceptual analysis of voice.[4] Developed in 1981, this scheme is not a complete perceptual evaluation protocol but specifically evaluates voice quality. It assesses the following:

- Grade (the overall degree of voice abnormality),
- Roughness (perceived irregularity in voicing source),
- Breathiness (audible air escape in voice),
- Asthenia (voice weakness), and
- Strain (perception of excessive vocal effort).

Each parameter is quantified on a 4-point scale, where 0 = normal, 1 = mild, 2 = moderate, and 3 = severe.[4] Another commonly used scheme is the Consensus Auditory-Perceptual Evaluation of Voice. Its primary purpose is to describe the severity of auditory-perceptual attributes of a voice problem, in a way that can be communicated among clinicians. Its secondary purpose is to contribute to hypotheses regarding the anatomic and physiologic bases of voice problems and to evaluate the need for additional testing.[6]

EXAMINATION

Typically, perceptual voice assessment is initiated before physical examination of the patient; the physician should already have a diagnostic inclination based on history and perceptual evaluation of voice. Abnormalities such as mucosal disturbance, glottic insufficiency, or a neurologic movement disorder are often suspected based solely on the initial history and voice assessment. Any major incongruity between this preliminary impression and subsequent laryngostroboscopic findings should serve as concern that the evaluation is incomplete.

HEAD AND NECK EXAMINATION

A full head and neck examination should be performed at the time of initial consultation. This should include assessment of motion and, where appropriate, symmetry of structures of the face, oral cavity, head, neck, and respiratory system. This should include a dedicated evaluation of external laryngeal anatomy and extrinsic laryngeal musculature.

An assessment of respiration is of particular relevance in order to evaluate coordination of respiration with phonation. This assessment includes noting the respiratory pattern (abdominal, thoracic, clavicular), looking for breath-holding patterns, or any habitual use of residual air.

LARYNGEAL EXAMINATION

Indirect visualization of the larynx is the hallmark of in-office laryngological evaluation. It allows the clinician to make observations of laryngeal structure and function while the patient is awake and reasonably comfortable. For voice evaluation to be comprehensive it is imperative to understand both functional deviation and anatomic abnormalities noted on examination.

The larynx can be visualized using many different instruments. The most commonly used instruments are mirror, transnasal flexible fiberoptic endoscopy, and rigid transoral endoscopy. In modern times, the ability to record and document an examination is more meaningful than the ease and cost-effectiveness of the mirror examination. The patient is able to vocalize in a more natural fashion with fiberoptic endoscopy, thus making flexible or rigid videoendoscopy the current standard of assessment.

Videoendoscopy offers insight into structure and gross function of the larynx. It will show any evidence of supraglottic compression during sustained phonation. Moreover, it can evaluate movement of vocal folds during laryngeal tasks to give information on gross vocal fold mobility.[7] Certain factors may limit the utility of endoscopy. Image clarity may be suboptimal and patients may be uncomfortable, have anatomy that makes the examination more difficult, have anxiety about the test, or have a hypersensitive gag reflex.

FLEXIBLE LARYNGOSCOPY

The flexible fiberoptic laryngoscope is a valuable tool that is ubiquitously present for most, if not all, otolaryngologists. It is a well-tolerated examination and is easily performed by otolaryngologists and trainees. Although there are limitations to the examination, it can provide, at minimum, visualization of the vocal folds through continuous light. It is least disturbing to the production of speech, which makes it ideal for evaluation of neurogenic voice disorders. However, the low resolution and lack of magnification make the flexible fiberoptic laryngoscope suboptimal to view small mucosal lesions. Newer, contemporary, "chip-tip" laryngoscopes that do away with fibers provide a clearer picture, especially as imaging quality becomes of higher definition.

RIGID ENDOSCOPY

The rigid endoscope transmits images via a glass rod. Although this offers a higher resolution picture, it also requires an increased skill level by the examiner. It does, however, confer the diagnostic advantage of image quality and zoom to evaluate mucosal abnormalities. This is especially true when videostroboscopy is concurrently used.

STROBOSCOPY

Stroboscopy can be performed via flexible or rigid endoscopy and uses a pulsed light source synced to the patient's vocal frequency to give the illusion of a slow motion mucosal oscillation. It requires periodic vibration to capture oscillation. It confers the single best diagnostic instrument in most of the dysphonia cases and is oftentimes the only method of obtaining information on mucosal pliability. It functions by pulsing light at a frequency that is incongruent with the glottal cycle, thus generating a series of still images across different points of the glottal cycle.[2] This image seems fluid to the examiner's eye due to Talbot's law, which states that images presented more quickly than 200 ms (5 images per second) are seen as a constant, smoothly moving image.

Stroboscopy can provide information on the following components of the glottic cycle:

- Regularity: uniformity of sequential glottic cycles
- Amplitude: lateral movement of the vocal fold in the medial plane
- Mucosal wave: the movement of the mucosal cover of the vocal fold
- Phase symmetry: symmetry of the left compared with the right vocal fold with regard to opening, closing, medial to lateral excursion
- Vertical level: symmetry of the left and right vocal fold in the vertical plane
- Glottic closure: pattern of complete versus types of incomplete glottic closure patterns[7]

The standard of care in laryngoscopic evaluation and documentation involves video recording of these examinations. Stroboscopy also uses the video recording aspect to enhance the examination by slowing down the play-back to reveal aspects of pathology not initially seen. The physician can rewatch the examination in freeze-frame or slow motion to improve diagnostic accuracy. Moreover, video recording/archiving allows for comparison of examinations across time as well as before and after interventions. Stroboscopy can often delineate abnormalities that were not seen on initial fiberoptic endoscopy but were clearly present based on patient history and perceptual examination of the voice. Certain pathologic conditions, such as sulcus and alterations in mucosal pliability, are most reliably diagnosed with stroboscopy. Patients with malignant and premalignant vocal fold changes also benefit from stroboscopy because the physician can compare vascularity and mucosal pliability as part of routine surveillance pre- and posttreatment.

High-speed imaging and videokymography are 2 additional imaging modalities that allow for even higher definition evaluation of vocal fold vibration. High-speed videoendoscopy allows for true vibratory cycle evaluation in each vocal fold due to a dramatically higher frame per second image capture compared with videostroboscopy. It does not require periodic vibration and can evaluate a periodic vocal fold vibration that can be seen in pathology such as vocal fold scar. Videokymography is often a component of high-speed imaging. Videokymography evaluates the vocal folds via a horizontal plane through the glottis. The images derived allow for evaluation of left-right asymmetries, mucosal wave propagation, and glottic closure parameters. At present, these modalities offer great potential for enhanced understanding and evaluation of laryngeal biomechanics but remain relegated to research institutions due to expense and incompletely determined day to day clinical utility beyond videostroboscopy and high-definition endoscopy.

AERODYNAMIC ASSESSMENT

Aerodynamic assessment can be helpful to analyze vocal function. It involves measuring glottal aerodynamic parameters required for phonation, including subglottal pressure, airflow, and glottal efficiency.

Subglottal air pressure is necessary to sustain vocal fold vibration. In order to be assessed directly, pressure below the vocal folds would require a tracheal puncture. An estimate of this can be made by measuring intraoral pressure during a voiceless stop consonant. Subglottal air pressure varies widely based on age, gender, loudness, consonant tested, and speech context. Abnormal pressures can be secondary to velopharyngeal insufficiency, glottic insufficiency, inadequate pulmonary reserve, or changes in vocal fold stiffness.

Glottal airflow is commonly assessed during sustained phonation and is estimated from oral airflow rate during vowel production. It can be abnormal with poor glottic closure from any means, such as vocal fold motion impairment or mass effect.

Another important concept is maximum phonation time (MPT).[8] MPT can assess for glottic insufficiency, which may indicate laryngeal pathology. However, its limitation is extreme variability with the normal range for healthy young adults as 6.6 to 69.5 seconds.[8] Many factors influence MPT including respiratory capacity and function, phonatory function, resonance, practice, frequency, intensity, instructions, and vowel choice.[9] If MPT is used, it should be collected using standard instructions and coaching, and the longest of 3 trials should be reported.

An assessment of velopharyngeal airflow is helpful in determining presence of velopharyngeal competence, which can be estimated by intraoral air pressure and nasal airflow during stop consonants. In contrast, the presence of low intraoral air pressure and high nasal airflow during nonnasal consonants indicates velopharyngeal incompetence.[10] Speech pathologists with expertise in voice will be critical to performing the above testing.

SUMMARY

Each component of voice evaluation plays a critical role in painting the picture of the patient's voice disturbance. Any disparity between history, perceptual evaluation, and laryngoscopic examination should prompt further evaluation and workup. For example, a fiberoptic examination that does not reveal any pathology in the presence of vocal disruption should prompt further evaluation with stroboscopic evaluation.

The goal of voice evaluation is to comprehensively assess the voice. This may lead to the diagnosis of a voice disorder but at minimum involves a clinical description of the characteristics and severity of the disorder. Ultimately, it is the clinician's goal to provide recommendations for intervention with subsequent identification of appropriate treatment and management options. This often includes multidisciplinary management with speech and language pathologists, neurologists, gastroenterologists, and pulmonary specialists. It is the senior author's opinion that video archiving is also critical for surveillance of lesions over time and evaluation of posttreatment outcomes for vocal fold movement, closure, and biomechanics.

REFERENCES

1. Cummings CW. Voice evaluation and therapy. Otolaryngology – head and neck surgery. 6th edition. Philadelphia: Elsevier Mosby; 2015. p. 846–53.
2. Sulica L. Laryngoscopy, stroboscopy and other tools for the evaluation of voice disorders. Otolaryngol Clin North Am 2013;46(1):21–30.
3. Rosen CA, Lee AS, Osborne J, et al. Development and validation of the voice handicap index-10. Laryngoscope 2004;114:1549–56.
4. Hogikyan ND, Sethuraman G. Validation of an instrument to measure voice-related quality of life. J Voice 1999;13:557–69.
5. Back KK, Befalsky PC, Wayslil K, et al. Validity and reliability of the Glottal Function Index. Arch Otolaryngol Head Neck Surg 2005;131(11):961–4.
6. American Speech-Language-Hearing Association special interest division 3, voice and voice disorders. Consensus auditory perceptual evaluation of voice (CAPE-V). 2003. Available at: http://www.asha.org. Accessed October 1, 2018.

7. American Speech-Language-Hearing Association. Recommended protocols for instrumental assessment of voice. 2015. Available at: http://www.asha.org. Accessed October 1, 2018.
8. Speyer R, Bogaardt HC, Passos VL, et al. Maximum phonation time: variability and reliability. J Voice 2010;24:281–4.
9. Solomon NP, Garlitz SJ, Milbrath RL. Respiratory and laryngeal contributions to maximum phonation time. J Voice 2000;14:331.
10. Rieves AL, Regner MF, Jiang JJ. Phonation threshold pressure estimation using electroglottography in an airflow redirection system. Laryngoscope 2009;119: 2378–83.

Hoarseness Guidelines Redux

Toward Improved Treatment of Patients with Dysphonia

David O. Francis, MD, MS[a],*, Libby J. Smith, DO[b]

KEYWORDS

- Hoarseness • Dysphonia • Laryngitis • Guidelines • Laryngoscopy • Management

KEY POINTS

- Hoarseness and dysphonia are symptoms of an underlying condition that requires nuanced history and physical examination, including laryngoscopy, to properly diagnose.
- Escalation of care to include expedited laryngoscopy is essential when patients present with alarm signs or symptoms.
- Proton pump inhibitors and other antireflux medications, antimicrobials, and corticosteroids should not be prescribed to treat isolated hoarseness until after the larynx has been examined.
- A mainstay of treatment of hoarseness/dysphonia both before and after laryngeal examination should be educating patients about control and preventive measures.

INTRODUCTION

Clinical Practice Guidelines have been widely embraced in medicine, and Otolaryngology, as a specialty, was an early adopter. The field cares for some of the most common surgical and nonsurgical conditions in health care today, including hearing loss, otitis media, sinusitis, and tonsillitis. These conditions affect a large population of patients and are managed by many different medical specialties. It is therefore essential that associated clinical practice guidelines are developed in a multidisciplinary manner in order to optimize management decisions for these common conditions across specialties.

Disclosure Statement: The authors have nothing to disclose.
[a] Division of Otolaryngology–Head and Neck Surgery, Wisconsin Surgical Outcomes Research Program, Department of Surgery, University of Wisconsin – Madison, 600 Highland Avenue, K4/7, Madison, WI 53792-7375, USA; [b] Department of Otolaryngology–Head and Neck Surgery, University of Pittsburgh, Eye & Ear Institute, Suite 500, 203 Lothrop Street, Pittsburgh, PA 15213, USA
* Corresponding author.
E-mail address: dofrancis@wisc.edu

The Institute of Medicine specifies that "guidelines are systematically developed statements to assist practitioner and patient decisions about appropriate health care for specific clinical circumstances."[1] The impetus for guidelines is severalfold. First, they raise awareness of an important clinical problem. Second, they provide an evidence-based resource for clinicians and patients that is useful at the point of care. Third, guidelines are intended to reduce unnecessary variations in care that derive from uncertainty or lack of knowledge of best evidence. Uncertainty fosters higher health care costs and inefficient resource allocation and may result in poorer patient outcomes.[2]

The American Academy of Otolaryngology–Head and Neck Surgery (AAO-HNS) has created many condition-specific clinical practice guidelines (eg, otitis media with effusion,[3,4] allergic rhinitis,[4] adult sinusitis,[5] benign paroxysmal positional vertigo[6]), but also several guidelines focused on physical examination findings (eg, neck mass[7]), surgeries,[8,9] and symptoms.[10–12] The Hoarseness Guidelines represent an example that focuses on a symptom. Hoarseness has many causes, and recognition that someone is hoarse or dysphonic is insufficient to provide definitive treatment recommendations, because the underlying cause is unknown without further workup. Instead, the Hoarseness Guidelines outline how a clinician should approach a patient who presents with dysphonia by providing guidance on evaluation and management decisions. It was designed for all clinicians, including primary care physicians, who care for patients with hoarseness of any age from pediatric to elderly. Herein, the authors provide a summary and critique of the AAO-HNS guideline developmental process and discuss recommendations from the Hoarseness Guideline Update.

PROCESS

The AAO-HNS guideline process is well defined and documented and abides by international standards for guideline development.[13–15] In the case of these guidelines, an information specialist performed a review of several databases and platforms (eg, PubMed search, CINAHL, National Guideline Clearinghouse) based on broad search terms (eg, dysphonia, hoarseness, voice disorder, laryngitis) and used a validated filter strategy to identify relevant (a) clinical practice guidelines, (b) systematic reviews, and (c) randomized controlled trials published since the original guideline.[10,11] This process ultimately yielded 3 new clinical practice guidelines, 16 systematic reviews, and 4 randomized controlled trials related to dysphonia.

This guideline developmental process has limitations. First and foremost is that the literature on dysphonia and hoarseness rarely includes the types of studies that the search strategy was designed to find, namely, rigorous controlled studies. Most related studies are of lower quality evidence, which does not necessarily mean they are less important. Moreover, dysphonia research is not monolithic; rather, this literature overlaps with several different subtopics (eg, reflux, antibiotic use, diagnostic modalities). By not performing a systematic review for each key action statement (KAS) risks, the literature review risks omitting important studies about a particular topic.

GUIDELINE RECOMMENDATIONS

Many KAS remained the same from the Initial Hoarseness Guidelines.[10,11] However, a few were added de novo or substantively altered based on newly available evidence. The authors discuss and interpret each KAS in the following discussion (**Table 1**).

Initial Presentation

Most otolaryngologists recognize that hoarseness is the description of voice change shared by a presenting patient and that dysphonia is the medical description of this

Table 1
Clinical practice guideline: hoarseness (dysphonia) (update) key action statements and strength of each recommendation

Key Action Statement	Strength
1 Clinicians should identify dysphonia in a patient with altered voice quality, pitch, loudness, or vocal effort that impairs communication or reduces quality of life	Recommendation
2 Clinicians should assess the patient with dysphonia by history and physical examination for underlying causes of dysphonia and factors that modify management	Recommendation
3 Clinicians should assess the patient with dysphonia by history and physical examination to identify factors whereby expedited laryngeal evaluation is indicated	Strong recommendation
4a Clinicians may perform diagnostic laryngoscopy at any time in a patient with dysphonia	Option
4b Clinicians should perform laryngoscopy, or refer to a clinician who can perform laryngoscopy, when dysphonia fails to resolve or improve within 4 wk or irrespective of duration if a serious underlying cause is suspected	Recommendation
5 Clinicians should not obtain computed tomography or MRI for patients with a primary voice complaint before visualization of the larynx	Recommendation against
6 Clinicians should not prescribe antireflux medications to treat isolated dysphonia, based on symptoms alone attributed to suspected gastroesophageal reflux disease or laryngopharyngeal reflux, without visualization of the larynx	Recommendation against
7 Clinicians should not routinely prescribe corticosteroids for patients with dysphonia before visualization of the larynx	Recommendation against
8 Clinicians should not routinely prescribe antibiotics to treat dysphonia	Strong recommendation against
9a Clinicians should perform laryngoscopy, or refer to a clinician who can perform diagnostic laryngoscopy, before prescribing voice therapy and document/communicate the results to the speech-language pathologist	Recommendation
9b Clinicians should advocate voice therapy for patients with dysphonia from a cause amenable to voice therapy	Strong recommendation
10 Clinicians should advocate for surgery as a therapeutic option for patients with dysphonia with conditions amenable to surgical intervention	Recommendation
11 Clinicians should offer, or refer to clinician who can offer, botulinum toxin injections for the treatment of dysphonia caused by spasmodic dysphonia and other types of laryngeal dystonia	Recommendation
12 Clinicians should inform patients with dysphonia about control/preventive measures	Recommendation
13 Clinicians should document resolution, improvement, or worsened symptoms of dysphonia or change in quality of life among patients with dysphonia after treatment or observation	Recommendation

Adapted from Stachler RJ, Francis DO, Schwartz SR, et al. Clinical practice guideline: hoarseness (Dysphonia) (Update). Otolaryngol Head Neck Surg 2018;158 (1_suppl):S8; with permission.

symptom. This distinction is *KAS #1*, which did not change with this update. Regardless of the nomenclature used (hoarseness vs dysphonia), both describe a *symptom* of an underlying disease process. The reason this statement is considered important is that clinicians should not ignore dysphonia, regardless of whether they are evaluating patients for other issues, because it may herald a more serious underlying disease.

Similarly, *KAS #2* seems quite obvious; namely, perform a history and physical examination to evaluate the underlying cause of the voice change. Taking an appropriate history to identify potential causes of dysphonia is nuanced. The associated discussion within the guideline is designed to help all clinicians to tailor their history and physical examination in order to develop an informed differential diagnosis from which to form a management plan. Assumptions are too often made (eg, "it must be reflux"), in part, because insufficient time is taken to really understand the multitude of factors that may be contributing to patients' dysphonia.

These sentiments directly motivated the addition of *KAS #3* to this update, which relates to identifying situations whereby escalation of care is indicated. Escalation of care means expediently referring patients with alarm symptoms or extraordinary circumstances for specialist laryngeal examination. However, in order to recognize alarm symptoms, they must be elicited in the patient history and physical examination (*KAS #2*). Strong evidence exists that early referral to an otolaryngologist is indicated if a patient is experiencing dysphonia *and* stridor, has a concomitant neck mass, has a history of smoking, has a recent history of anterior head, neck, or chest surgery, was recently intubated, has unexplained weight loss, dysphagia, or concomitant neurologic symptoms (eg, dysarthria), among others. Head and neck cancer is perhaps the most time-sensitive diagnosis, because it may insidiously present first with nonspecific dysphonia. Identifying alarm symptoms and early referral in patients with concerning features can result in better patient outcomes.

Many otolaryngologists minimize the importance of this *KAS #3*, again, feeling that it is intended for other types of clinicians because awareness of alarm symptoms and appropriate triage is already part of their standard practice. All clinicians, including experienced otolaryngologists who care for patients with dysphonia, may overlook these alarm symptoms if they are not careful. In some situations, a simple laryngoscopy can uncover or refute a serious cause. However, when the clinical scenario remains unclear, it is often necessary to refer to a laryngologist and speech language pathology team that can perform and properly interpret videostroboscopy and other advanced diagnostic tests that may provide necessary data to make an informed diagnosis and treatment plan.

LARYNGEAL EXAMINATION

It is the authors' opinion that anyone presenting with dysphonia to a clinician should have a laryngeal examination. Historically, all clinicians were trained to perform indirect mirror laryngoscopy as part of the standard physical examination. Mirror laryngoscopy is an ideal tool to initially screen patients with hoarseness. Unfortunately, few current practitioners (otolaryngologists included) are facile with laryngeal mirror examination. Thus, laryngoscopy has become the domain of the otolaryngologist and is done, most often, using transnasal flexible laryngoscopes. This has important implications for the Hoarseness Guidelines and has particular relevance for *KAS #4*, which has 2 parts. The first part (a) states that laryngoscopy may be performed at any time in a patient with dysphonia. It is not the intention of the guideline to limit the autonomy of clinicians to perform any physical examination that they feel is necessary and relevant. However, more than 95% of all patients with dysphonia are cared for by nonotolaryngologists who do not have the training nor the ability to perform laryngos-copy.[16,17] It is incumbent on the otolaryngology community to provide guidance to these referring providers, as to when it is appropriate to advocate that patients have a formal laryngeal examination. This rationale was the impetus for the second part of *KAS #4* (b), which states that any patient whose dysphonia fails to resolve within 4 weeks should be referred for laryngoscopy or irrespective of duration if a serious un-derlying cause is suspected. The time period recommended was significantly changed from the original guideline that recommended referral if dysphonia persisted more than 3 months.[10] The former timeframe was controversial and was revised in the update based on new evidence.[18] A 3-month timeframe was considered too long, because delaying evaluation for a potentially serious underlying cause could result in higher initial cancer staging, need for more aggressive treatments, and prolonging of serious quality-of-life consequences.[19] If the diagnosis remains unclear after transnasal or transoral laryngoscopy, then escalation of care to a laryngologist is advisable.

"LOOK BEFORE YOU ACT" MANAGEMENT

The next 4 KAS refer to what are appropriate management decisions for patients who have acute (<4 weeks) hoarseness without any alarm symptoms or circumstances. These statements have caused many in the community to refer to this as the *"Guide-line of No."* However, all the following statements are based on strong evidence and are designed to deescalate and prevent inappropriate use of resources and to mini-mize potential harm to patients and, transitively, the entire population.

KAS #5 relates to imaging for dysphonia. The risk of harm and absence of benefit to imaging the larynx before performing laryngoscopy is clear. Radiation is not benign and should not be used or advocated for in patients with acute hoarseness before they have a visual laryngeal examination. This statement did not change with the up-date and is widely agreed on in the otolaryngology community. Nonetheless and despite the evidence, the authors often are referred patients who have had unneces-sary computed tomography scans, which could have been avoided if these patients had simply been referred directly for laryngoscopy.

KAS #6 relates to antireflux medication and dysphonia; namely that "clinicians should not prescribe antireflux medications to treat isolated dysphonia, based on symptoms alone attributed to suspected gastroesophageal reflux disease or laryngo-pharyngeal reflux, without visualizing the larynx." The message of this KAS is manifold. First, it argues against empiric treatment of *isolated* hoarseness with antireflux medi-cation by providers who have not first evaluated the larynx. Unfortunately, many pa-tients presenting to the authors' clinics with hoarseness have been trialed on or are currently on proton pump inhibitors (PPI) medication despite overwhelming data from placebo-controlled randomized controlled trials showing no effect on isolated hoarseness. Unfortunately, this practice pattern has seeped into the mainstream[20,21] and needs to be corrected.

The purpose of this statement is not to imply that reflux cannot cause hoarseness, but rather that before starting the patient on a PPI, a clinician should look at the larynx and make sure there is not an alternative explanation for their symptoms.[22–24] Symp-toms commonly attributed to reflux are vague and can have many explanations (eg, globus, throat irritation). *Look before you prescribe is a good rule.* It is also important for the greater otolaryngology community to know that laryngoscopy alone is insuffi-cient to diagnose laryngopharyngeal reflux despite historical arguments to the con-trary.[25–28] Recent studies have consistently shown this, and the practice of making "definitive" reflux diagnoses based on laryngoscopy is discouraged. Patients with hoarseness without a clear explanation even after careful laryngeal examination may be placed on a course of PPI therapy with the understanding that if it is not effective, then acid reflux is either not the culprit or further diagnostic testing is indicated.

KAS #7 recommends against empiric treatment of dysphonia with corticosteroids before a laryngeal examination is performed. This recommendation is based on strong evidence showing harm and little benefit to use of empiric steroids. As a general rule, in a patient with hoarseness, absent a laryngeal examination, it is not clear what is being treated. Steroids are not benign and have many well-documented side effects. Although they may reduce inflammation, using them without knowledge of the underlying laryngeal disease being treated may ultimately be injurious to the patient while also delaying appropriate diagnosis and treatment. The guideline panel unanimously agreed that empiric use of steroids for isolated dysphonia is not advisable. It is important to clarify that steroid can be a helpful adjunct to treatment,[24] but only after a proper laryngeal examination has been performed and the clinical situation is appropriate.

KAS #8 is based on clear level I, randomized controlled trial evidence that argues against clinicians routinely prescribing antibiotics to treat dysphonia.[29] Recommendation might seem obvious to otolaryngologists; however, it is still common practice for many health care practitioners.[30] Patients often present to clinics stating that "my doctor prescribed an antibiotic and steroids" for their hoarseness, invariably without examining the larynx. To be fair, there are circumstances in which antimicrobials and antifungals are indicated for bacterial and fungal laryngitis, respectively. However, these are few and far between when the totality of patients with hoarseness is considered. Individualized patient care is required, but antimicrobials should not be considered a routine, empiric treatment for isolated dysphonia without some corroborating physical examination findings, which requires laryngoscopy and potentially culture. The consequences of antibiotic resistance are stark, and the role in preventing the furtherance of this epidemic should not be underestimated.

"AFTER YOU LOOK" MANAGEMENT

Definitive diagnosis and treatment of dysphonic patients whose symptoms do not spontaneously resolve within 4 weeks or have alarm symptoms necessitate careful laryngeal examination. Once a diagnosis has been made (or presumed) based on laryngoscopy, treatment options may include voice therapy, medical management, surgery, physical therapy, and education, either as monotherapies or in combination. *KAS #9* relates to voice therapy, which is a stalwart treatment for many types of dysphonia. The statement has 2 parts (a, b). First, laryngoscopy by a clinician should be performed before voice therapy in patients with dysphonia. This laryngoscopy is to ensure that there is a discrete diagnosis that is being treated. It is a well-established practice to ensure proper communication between clinicians and speech-language pathologists and to ensure that the condition diagnosed is, in fact, amenable to voice therapy. Some acute and most chronic voice conditions benefit from combined clinician and speech-language pathology input. Voice therapy can be a primary treatment, as in the case of muscle tension dysphonia, or may be adjunctive to medical or surgical treatment (eg, glottal insufficiency). Accordingly, *KAS #9(b)* states that clinicians should advocate for voice therapy in patients with dysphonia from causes amenable to voice therapy.

KAS #10 focuses on surgery. Laryngoscopy or videostroboscopy is essential to identify underlying causes of dysphonia in which surgery may be an option. Examples include malignancy/premalignancy, benign vocal fold lesions that do not respond to conservative management, glottal insufficiency, and papilloma. Surgical treatment is often performed in conjunction with adjunctive preoperative or postoperative voice therapy, which can play a critical rehabilitative role. There are many potential surgical indications for voice-related conditions, but it behooves all surgeons to be contemplative in selecting only those patients who are likely to benefit. Surgery has well-known risks and benefits, and many conditions that 20 years ago were thought to be primarily surgical are now almost universally treated with conservative therapy (eg, nodules). The clinician's role is to educate the patient about surgical options and to make shared, informed decisions about the best approach for each patient's situation.

A distinct set of patients with spasmodic dysphonia or other laryngeal dystonia has been shown to benefit from botulinum toxin into intrinsic laryngeal muscles. *KAS #11* states that clinicians should offer, or refer to someone who can offer, botulinum toxin injections for the treatment of dysphonia caused by spasmodic dysphonia and other laryngeal dystonias. These conditions are debilitating, but patients receiving regular botulinum injections can experience improvement in voice such that they can communicate effectively in most settings and function in society. Although botulinum toxin for this indication is not currently Food and Drug Administration approved, it is approved by the Center for Medicare and Medicaid Services based on the preponderance of benefit over harm.

KAS #12 is perhaps the most important of all statements because it has relevance at each stage ("Before You Look" and "After You Look") and presentation of patients with dysphonia. It states that clinicians should inform patients with dysphonia about control and preventive measures. This approach should be the primary management for acute dysphonia (<4 weeks) because it has the potential to promote symptom resolution without any intervention. It is also important to teach patients who are prone to dysphonia how to mitigate their propensity for recurrence. Examples of educational materials that would benefit patients with dysphonia are included within the main dysphonia guideline publication[11] and further developed in the plain language summary.[31]

The last statement, *KAS #13*, was added with the guideline update. It states that clinicians should document resolution, improvement, or worsened symptoms of dysphonia or change in quality of life among patients with dysphonia after treatment or observation. This may seem somewhat obvious, but is an often overlooked part of patient care. After starting any treatment or caring for a patient with watchful waiting, it is important that it is documented how the patient fared with the treatment decisions. If there is no improvement or worsened symptoms that are either concerning or affecting quality of life, then repeat evaluation or referral to a specialist (laryngologist) is probably indicated. Documenting outcomes of treatments should be compulsory. It is essential to continually improve patient care while demonstrating treatments are effective to regulatory agencies, especially in the current health care environment.

SUMMARY

The guideline update provides an evidence-based approach to patients presenting to the clinic with hoarseness that is applicable to all clinicians who care for this population. It reviews the management decisions in acute and chronic dysphonia and before and after laryngeal examination. In general, medical and surgical interventions should not be offered until the larynx has been examined. The guidance offered is designed to aid all clinicians regardless of specialty in providing the best possible evidence-based care for patients presenting with dysphonia.

REFERENCES

1. Institute of Medicine Committee on Standards for Developing Trustworthy Clinical Practice Guidelines. In: Graham R, Mancher M, Miller Wolman D, et al, editors.

Clinical practice guidelines we can trust. Washington, DC: National Academies Press (US); 2011. Copyright 2011 by the National Academy of Sciences. All rights reserved.

2. Birkmeyer JD, Reames BN, McCulloch P, et al. Understanding of regional variation in the use of surgery. Lancet 2013;382(9898):1121–9.

3. Rosenfeld RM, Shin JJ, Schwartz SR, et al. Clinical practice guideline: otitis media with effusion (update). Otolaryngol Head Neck Surg 2016;154(1 Suppl): S1–41.

4. Seidman MD, Gurgel RK, Lin SY, et al. Clinical practice guideline: allergic rhinitis. Otolaryngol Head Neck Surg 2015;152(1 Suppl):S1–43.

5. Rosenfeld RM, Piccirillo JF, Chandrasekhar SS, et al. Clinical practice guideline (update): adult sinusitis. Otolaryngol Head Neck Surg 2015;152(2 Suppl):S1–39.

6. Bhattacharyya N, Baugh RF, Orvidas L, et al. Clinical practice guideline: benign paroxysmal positional vertigo. Otolaryngol Head Neck Surg 2008;139(5 Suppl 4): S47–81.

7. Pynnonen MA, Gillespie MB, Roman B, et al. Clinical practice guideline: evaluation of the neck mass in adults. Otolaryngol Head Neck Surg 2017;157(2_suppl): S1–30.

8. Baugh RF, Archer SM, Mitchell RB, et al. Clinical practice guideline: tonsillectomy in children. Otolaryngol Head Neck Surg 2011;144(1 Suppl):S1–30.

9. Rosenfeld RM, Schwartz SR, Pynnonen MA, et al. Clinical practice guideline: tympanostomy tubes in children. Otolaryngol Head Neck Surg 2013;149(1 Suppl): S1–35.

10. Schwartz SR, Cohen SM, Dailey SH, et al. Clinical practice guideline: hoarseness (dysphonia). Otolaryngol Head Neck Surg 2009;141(3 Suppl 2):S1–31.

11. Stachler RJ, Francis DO, Schwartz SR, et al. Clinical practice guideline: hoarseness (dysphonia) (update). Otolaryngol Head Neck Surg 2018;158(1_suppl): S1–42.

12. Tunkel DE, Bauer CA, Sun GH, et al. Clinical practice guideline: tinnitus. Otolaryngol Head Neck Surg 2014;151(2 Suppl):S1–40.

13. Rosenfeld RM, Shiffman RN, Robertson P. Clinical practice guideline development manual, third edition: a quality-driven approach for translating evidence into action. Otolaryngol Head Neck Surg 2013;148(1 Suppl):S1–55.

14. Methods guide for effectiveness and comparative effectiveness reviews. AHRQ Publication No. 10(14)-EHC063-EF. Rockville, MD: Agency for Healthcare Research and Quality. 2014. Available at: http://www.effectivehealthcare.ahrq. gov. Accessed May 7, 2019.

15. American Academy of Pediatrics Steering Committee on Quality improvement and Management. Classifying recommendations for clinical practice guidelines. Pediatrics 2004;114(3):874–7.

16. Cohen SM, Kim J, Roy N, et al. Factors influencing referral of patients with voice disorders from primary care to otolaryngology. Laryngoscope 2014;124(1): 214–20.

17. Cohen SM, Kim J, Roy N, et al. Delayed otolaryngology referral for voice disorders increases health care costs. Am J Med 2015;128(4):426.e11-8.

18. Cohen SM, Lee HJ, Roy N, et al. Chronicity of voice-related health care utilization in the general medicine community. Otolaryngol Head Neck Surg 2017;156(4): 693–701.

19. Chen AY, Halpern M. Factors predictive of survival in advanced laryngeal cancer. Arch Otolaryngol Head Neck Surg 2007;133(12):1270–6.

20. Ruiz R, Jeswani S, Andrews K, et al. Hoarseness and laryngopharyngeal reflux: a survey of primary care physician practice patterns. JAMA Otolaryngol Head Neck Surg 2014;140(3):192–6.
21. Dion G, Amin MR, Branski RC. Treating hoarseness with proton pump inhibitors. JAMA 2015;314(12):1294–5.
22. Francis DO, Vaezi MF. Should the reflex be reflux? Throat symptoms and alternative explanations. Clin Gastroenterol Hepatol 2015;13(9):1560–6.
23. Sulica L. Hoarseness misattributed to reflux: sources and patterns of error. Ann Otol Rhinol Laryngol 2014;123(6):442–5.
24. Rafii B, Taliercio S, Achlatis S, et al. Incidence of underlying laryngeal pathology in patients initially diagnosed with laryngopharyngeal reflux. Laryngoscope 2014; 124(6):1420–4.
25. Fritz MA, Persky MJ, Fang Y, et al. The accuracy of the laryngopharyngeal reflux diagnosis: utility of the stroboscopic exam. Otolaryngol Head Neck Surg 2016; 155(4):629–34.
26. Hicks DM, Ours TM, Abelson TI, et al. The prevalence of hypopharynx findings associated with gastroesophageal reflux in normal volunteers. J Voice 2002; 16(4):564–79.
27. Milstein CF, Charbel S, Hicks DM, et al. Prevalence of laryngeal irritation signs associated with reflux in asymptomatic volunteers: impact of endoscopic technique (rigid vs. flexible laryngoscope). Laryngoscope 2005;115(12):2256–61.
28. Powell J, Cocks HC. Mucosal changes in laryngopharyngeal reflux–prevalence, sensitivity, specificity and assessment. Laryngoscope 2013;123(4):985–91.
29. Reveiz L, Cardona AF. Antibiotics for acute laryngitis in adults. Cochrane Database Syst Rev 2015;(5):CD004783.
30. Cohen SM, Kim J, Roy N, et al. Assessing factors related to the pharmacologic management of laryngeal diseases and disorders. Laryngoscope 2013;123(7): 1763–9.
31. Krouse HJ, Reavis CCW, Stachler RJ, et al. Plain language summary: hoarseness (dysphonia). Otolaryngol Head Neck Surg 2018;158(3):427–31.

Identification and Management of Chronic Laryngitis

Alisa Zhukhovitskaya, MD, Sunil P. Verma, MD*

KEYWORDS

- Chronic laryngitis • Dysphonia • Hoarseness • Globus sensation • Cough

KEY POINTS

- There are many various infectious, inflammatory, and autoimmune causes of chronic laryngitis.
- Symptoms of various causes are usually nonspecific with a broad range of severity.
- Some causes of chronic laryngitis may mimic the appearance of carcinoma; biopsy allows differentiation between carcinoma and a benign cause of chronic laryngitis.

INTRODUCTION

Chronic laryngitis is defined as an inflammatory process of at least 3-week duration that encompasses a broad range of inflammatory, infectious, and autoimmune conditions resulting in alteration of phonation, breathing, and swallowing.[1] The incidence of chronic laryngitis is not well established but has been estimated as 3.47 diagnoses per 1000 people per year.[2] Symptoms are typically nonspecific and include dysphonia, throat pain, globus sensation, frequent throat clearing, cough, and dysphagia.[2] This article describes various causes of chronic laryngitis.

INFECTIOUS CAUSES OF CHRONIC LARYNGITIS
Bacterial Infections

Most bacterial laryngitis are acute; chronic bacterial laryngitis is suspected in patients with prolonged voice changes and laryngeal exudates and crusting despite attempted treatment of other causes of chronic laryngitis. Endoscopic findings include edema, erythema, and possible alterations in vocal fold vibration. Methicillin-susceptible and methicillin-resistant *Staphylococcus aureus* are the most common causative

Disclosure Statement: The authors have nothing to disclose.
Department of Otolaryngology–Head and Neck Surgery, University of California, Irvine, 101 The City Drive South, Building 56, Suite 500, Orange, CA 92868, USA
* Corresponding author.
E-mail address: verma@uci.edu

organisms; *Pseudomonas aeruginosa* and *Serratia marcescens* have also been reported.[3,4] Biofilms have been found in patients with chronic laryngitis and may act as pathogen reservoirs and explain relapses in symptoms after appropriate antibiotic treatment.[5] Purulent bacterial chondritis of the laryngeal framework may result from superinfection of prior laryngeal injury by *S aureus*. Symptoms include stridor, dyspnea, and dysphonia. Supraglottic edema and airway narrowing may be seen. Computed tomography (CT) with contrast may demonstrate edema of laryngeal cartilages, airways narrowing, and abscess formation. Treatment includes antibiotics, incision and drainage of abscesses, and tracheostomy in cases of airway compromise.[6]

Rhinoscleroma is a chronic granulomatous infection caused by *Klebsiella rhinoscleromatis*. It is endemic to the tropics and subtropics and typically affects the nose causing purulent rhinorrhea, atrophy, crusting, and granuloma formation. Laryngotracheal manifestations range from mild dysphonia to stridor, dyspnea, and respiratory compromise. Positive culture is diagnostic; typical histopathologic findings include Russell bodies and Mikulicz cells. Supraglottic, glottic, and subglottic granulomas as well as glottic and subglottic stenosis have been reported. Laryngoscopy exhibits pale lesions with diffuse nodular thickening. Treatment consists of tetracycline antibiotics, excision of discrete symptomatic lesions, subglottic dilation, and tracheostomy.[7]

Mycobacterial Infections

Mycobacterium tuberculosis most often causes chronic pulmonary infections with possible spread to other sites; primary tuberculosis of the larynx is rare. Patients typically complain of dysphonia, but may also experience odynophagia, dysphagia, coughing, and rarely dyspnea.[8] Laryngoscopy demonstrates generalized mucosal edema and hyperemia or discrete ulcerative or exophytic lesions, which may be solitary or multiple. Lesions most frequently affect the true vocal folds but may involve the ventricles, false vocal folds, epiglottis, and interarytenoid areas.[9] Laryngeal tuberculosis may be mistaken for carcinoma; biopsy helps differentiate the disorders. Histology may demonstrate giant cell granulomas with caseating necrosis. Purified protein derivative (PPD) may be negative in isolated laryngeal tuberculosis.[8] Given the high likelihood of concurrent pulmonary disease, obtaining a chest radiograph is essential.[9] Treatment consists of a combination of antimycobacterial drugs, including isoniazid, rifampin, and pyrazinamide for approximately 6 months.[8]

Dimorphic Fungal Infections

Blastomyces, *Paracoccidioides*, *Coccidioides*, and *Histoplasma* are dimorphic fungi; they exist in hyphal form in the environment and convert to pathogenic yeast form after entering a mammalian host. Infection occurs via inhalation; therefore the organisms initially cause pulmonary disease. Immunocompetent hosts may be asymptomatic or exhibit influenza-like symptoms; the disease is more severe in immunocompromised patients. The infection may disseminate to extrapulmonary sites, including the larynx, and also cause constitutional symptoms.[10] Systemic mycoses may be initially misdiagnosed on laryngoscopy as laryngeal carcinoma, given their rarity and similarity of appearance on laryngoscopy, as well as their similar symptoms; diagnosis typically requires biopsy and special tissue stains.[11–15] Infection should be suspected in patients with history of travel or residence in endemic regions, particularly if pulmonary symptoms are present.[10] Treatment consists of Amphotericin B and other antifungals.[13–17]

Blastomycosis

Blastomyces dermatitidis infections of the head and neck most often affect the larynx. The organism is endemic to the Midwest, Southwest, and South-Central United States and Canadian provinces adjacent to the Great Lakes. It may present as progressive hoarseness and possibly hemoptysis.[16] Exophytic or verrucous polypoid masses or ulceration and diffuse erythema may be visualized on the true and false vocal folds; true vocal folds may be hypomobile.[16,18] Histology demonstrates epithelial atypical and pseudoepitheliomatous hyperplasia, and possible giant cells and microabscesses; broad-based budding yeasts may be identified on Grocott methenamine silver (GMS) stain.[16,18] After treatment, patients may have persistent dysphonia, laryngeal stenosis, or chronic inflammatory changes.[16]

Paracoccidioidomycosis

Paracoccidioides brasiliensis is endemic to South America; laryngeal symptoms include dysphonia, dyspnea, dysphagia, and cough.[13] Lesions occur in any subunit of the larynx and may be multiple; laryngoscopy findings include ulceration, diffuse erythema, and exophytic mulberry-like lesions. Histology may demonstrate epitheliomatous hyperplasia, multinucleated giant cells, inflammatory cells, and round double-contoured budding organisms; a GMS stain may aid the diagnosis.[12,13]

Coccidioidomycosis

Coccidioides immitis is endemic to the Southwestern United States and parts of Central and South America.[11] Laryngeal infections present with throat soreness, dysphonia, and dyspnea.[11,17] The disease presents with granulomatous changes in any subunit of the larynx, erosion, diffuse erythema, and edema, or a fungating granuloma.[11,17]

Histoplasmosis

Histoplasma capsulatum chronic laryngitis is rare condition with fewer than 100 cases reported.[19] It is endemic to the Ohio and Mississippi River Valleys and has been reported in Latin American and Africa. Patients present with hoarseness, dysphagia, cough, stridor, and sore throat.[14,15,19] The larynx may demonstrate pearly white and edematous lesions, inflammation, painful ulcers, or submucosal masses.[14,19] Histology may demonstrate granulomatous lesions with foamy macrophages with intracellular organisms appearing as round or oval organisms surrounded by a clear zone, giant cells, plasma cells, lymphocytes, and necrosis.[15,19]

Cryptococcosis

Cryptococcus neoformans is a yeast that typically causes pulmonary infections in immunocompromised patients. Primary laryngeal cryptococcosis is uncommon and may present with dysphonia, dysphagia, and odynophagia. Laryngoscopy may demonstrate exudative or exophytic lesions, edema, and erythema. It may be mistaken clinically for carcinoma. Histology demonstrates inflammation, pseudoepitheliomatous hyperplasia; encapsulated oval-shaped budding yeast may be visualized on GMS stain. Treatment is with antifungals such as fluconazole.[20]

Viral Chronic Laryngitis

Herpes simplex virus

Herpes simplex virus chronic laryngitis is rare. It may present with dysphonia, dyspnea, dysphagia, or respiratory compromise. Laryngoscopy may demonstrate edema, ulceration of laryngeal mucosa, and exudates. Treatment is typically acyclovir.[21]

INFLAMMATORY CAUSES OF CHRONIC LARYNGITIS
Laryngopharyngeal Reflux

Laryngopharyngeal reflux is a common cause of chronic laryngitis; however, its pathophysiology, diagnosis, prevalence, and optimal treatment are controversial.[22] It is thought to be caused by incompetence or transient relaxation of lower esophageal sphincter resulting in retrograde flow of acid, pepsin, and possibly bile salts. This results either in direct pharyngeal and laryngeal mucosal damage or vagal stimulation in the distal esophagus.[22,23] Symptoms are nonspecific and include dysphonia, dysphagia, laryngospasm, throat discomfort, and choking sensation. Globus sensation, cough, and throat clearing may be particularly useful in diagnosis.[24,25] pH monitoring, laryngoscopy findings, empirical treatment with proton pump inhibitors (PPIs), and patient questionnaires have all been used for diagnosis.[22] Laryngoscopy may demonstrate erythema, diffuse or localized edema, cobble-stoning, excessive mucus, posterior commissure hypertrophy, vocal fold granuloma, and ventricular obliteration.[24,25] Treatment involves lifestyle modification, medication, and surgery.[22,24] Pharmacologic therapy consists of PPIs and less commonly H2-blocker; prokinetic agents have also been used.[22,23] PPIs may be used empirically for both treatment and confirmation of the diagnosis. Duration of treatment, dosing, outcome measures, and treatment of patients who fail PPIs are controversial.[23,25]

Idiopathic Ulcerative Laryngitis

Idiopathic ulcerative laryngitis presents as dysphonia and cough after a prolonged upper or lower respiratory infection. Laryngoscopic findings consist of bilateral ulceration of the midmembranous vocal folds. The condition is unresponsive to medical management; resolution of ulceration and improvement in dysphonia occurs within 2 to 4 months.[26]

Laryngitis Sicca

Laryngitis sicca is a poorly defined condition characterized by excessive dryness of the larynx, which may lead to significant crusting of laryngeal tissues. It has been proposed that the pathophysiology is similar to xerostomia.[27] Patients may present with throat clearing, sensation of throat dryness, and dysphonia.[28] Laryngitis sicca may result in keratinization of the vocal fold margin, stiffening of the vocal fold edge, and mass effect on the vocal folds; intraarytenoid area may exhibit pachydermia and the supraglottis may seem erythematous and friable.[29,30] Dehydration, tobacco use, noxious fumes, radiation, medication, or pollution may all be implicated in the condition.[29] Examples of medication are diazide, theophylline, steroid inhalers, and medications with anticholinergic effects that may promote mucosal drying.[28] Patients on anticholinergic medication have been shown to have a greater risk of complaining of hoarseness; the risk is even higher with multiple anticholinergic medications. These antimuscarinic medications have the effect of blocking acetylcholine release at nerve junctions that normally stimulate mucus-secreting glands. Increased viscosity of laryngeal mucus, which occurs with aging, may also contribute to the condition.[28] Treatment involves eliminating the underlying cause of laryngeal dryness.

Allergic Laryngitis

Allergic laryngitis is a controversial cause of chronic laryngitis; it may be misdiagnosed as laryngopharyngeal reflux given the overlap in symptoms.[31,32] Patients may demonstrate thick laryngeal secretions, transient vocal fold edema, erythema, and hyperemia resulting in voice changes, globus sensation, and frequent throat clearing. Allergic laryngitis may relate to the concept of a unified airway: upper and lower airways share common mediators and epithelial responses—stimulation at one site of the pathway may lead to sequelae in another (eg, immunoglobulin E (IgE)-mediated allergic reactions).[31] Support for existence of allergic laryngitis comes from epidemiologic studies showing increased voice symptoms in patients with allergic rhinitis and studies demonstrating a laryngeal response after stimulation with an allergen.[32] Allergy workup is indicated if allergic laryngitis is suspected, particularly if thick endolaryngeal mucus is present.[31,32]

SYSTEMIC INFLAMMATORY DISORDERS
Sarcoidosis

Sarcoidosis is a multisystem chronic inflammatory disorder of unknown cause; it most commonly affects the lungs and skin. Laryngeal involvement occurs in less than 5% but may be underdiagnosed given that not every patient undergoes laryngeal evaluation.[33,34] Patients present with hoarseness, throat pain, dysphagia, globus sensation, dyspnea, and stridor.[35,36] The disease most frequently affects the supraglottis, particularly the epiglottis; however the glottis and subglottis may also be involved.[33,34,36] Pathognomonic findings include edematous, pale, and diffusely enlarged supraglottis and "turbanlike" rounded appearance of the edge of the epiglottis.[36] Laryngoscopy may also demonstrate discrete nodular or erythematous areas in the supraglottis and thickening and erythema of the vocal folds. Histology often shows noncaseating granulomas consisting mostly of epithelioid cells with giant cells, plasma cells, and lymphocytes; however, sometimes only nonspecific lymphocytic infiltration is seen; stains are negative for fungus and mycobacteria.[33,36] Further workup may include chest radiography, PPD, and blood and urine analyses, and serum angiotensin converting enzyme (ACE) levels. ACE has low sensitivity and specificity for sarcoidosis but levels may be used to monitor disease course. Sarcoidosis may progress or regress spontaneously. Treatment of symptomatic disease includes intralesional or systemic steroids, localized mass excision, low-dose radiation, and (anecdotally) topical steroids.[33] Submucosal resection with preservation and closure of overlying mucosa has been advocated in order to reduce scarring and fibrosis.[35]

Amyloidosis

Amyloidosis is a group of disorders characterized by extracellular deposition of proteinaceous debris (amyloid) in tissue disrupting normal structure and function; it may be primary or secondary to lymphoproliferative or chronic inflammatory disorders such as rheumatoid arthritis (RA), multiple myeloma, and extramedullary plasmacytoma.[37] The larynx is the most common head and neck site. It presents with nonspecific symptoms of dysphagia, dyspnea, and cough; dysphonia is the most common symptom.[37–40] The supraglottis, particularly the false vocal folds, is most commonly involved, although the glottis and subglottis may also be affected; lesions may be single or multiple.[39,40] On laryngoscopy, amyloidosis appears as yellow- or orange-hued nodular or diffuse submucosal deposits.[40] Biopsy is required for diagnosis; Congo Red staining of the deposits with subsequent apple-green birefringence under polarized light is pathognomonic.[38] CT may demonstrate marked thickening of larynx; deposits may have intermediate T1 signal intensity and low T2 signal intensity on MRI.[38] Treatment consists of symptom-directed surgical excision; many patients require multiple procedures, as symptoms recur.[39,40] Laryngeal amyloidosis is less likely than other forms to be associated with systemic disease; however, systemic workup is still prudent although guidelines are not established.[39,40] Workup may involve general blood, liver, and urine tests; assessment of serum and urine for light chains; cardiac assessment; and radiolabeled scans to evaluate for amyloid deposits throughout the body. Long-term follow-up is required given the slowly progressive nature of the disorder.[38,40]

AUTOIMMUNE CAUSES OF CHRONIC LARYNGITIS
Granulomatosis with Polyangiitis

Granulomatosis with polyangiitis (GPA), also known as Wegener granulomatosis, is characterized by small vessel vasculitis and necrotizing granulomatous inflammation. It primarily affects the respiratory tract and kidneys. Disease is systemic or limited to a single organ system. It may cause laryngeal or tracheal ulcers or subglottic stenosis; the latter may lead to significant airway compromise. Symptoms include dyspnea, stridor, cough, and hoarseness.[41] It should be suspected in patients with other otolaryngologic GPA manifestations, including septal perforation; crusting; bleeding; purulent secretions of the nasal cavity and paranasal sinuses; otologic findings including otitis media, otitis externa-like symptoms, oral mucosal ulcers and gingival hyperplasia; and swelling of the parotid or submandibular glands.[41,42] Biopsy demonstrates inflammation and only rarely granulomatosis and vasculitis.[42] Many patients test positive for antineutrophil cytoplasmic autoantibodies (cytoplasmic antineutrophil cytoplasmic antibodies are most common; perinuclear antineutrophil cytoplasmic antibodies may also be positive).[41] Subglottic stenosis may present in absence of disease activity elsewhere and is frequently unresponsive to systemic immunosuppression. Symptomatic relief can be achieved with dilation, resection, and intralesional steroids.[42]

Relapsing Polychondritis

Relapsing polychondritis affects cartilage and other proteoglycan-rich tissues in the inner ear, eyes, skin, heart, and blood vessels; chondritis alone is seen in one-third of cases. The disorder is rare (4.5–9 cases per million) and systemic constitutional symptoms may be present. Patients experience periods of flare and remission and 90% exhibit auricular involvement during the disease course. In the airway, the trachea and mainstem bronchi are most commonly affected, although chondritis may be isolated to the larynx. Laryngeal involvement presents with dysphonia, dyspnea, stridor, cough, choking, and tenderness overlying the laryngeal cartilages. Laryngoscopy may demonstrate mucosal inflammation and infiltration of cartilage.[43] Airway stenosis may be present and require emergency tracheostomy or laryngotracheal reconstruction.[44] Diagnosis is made clinically; biopsy is rarely performed but may demonstrate infiltration with inflammatory cells, degeneration of chondrocytes, fibrosis, granulation, and decrease of basophilic staining of cartilage matrix due to decreased proteoglycan content. Attenuation of cartilage and thickening of airway walls may be seen on CT at early stages with stenosis and cartilaginous destruction at later stages. Treatment is empiric, with the aim of preventing irreversible tissue damage. Nonsteroidal antiinflammatory drugs are used in mild disease. Steroids and disease-modifying antirheumatic drugs (DMARDs) are used in advanced disease.[43]

Rheumatoid Arthritis

RA primarily affects joints but may cause myositis, anemia, and ocular symptoms. Up to 88% of patients demonstrate laryngeal involvement consisting of cricoarytenoid joint arthritis, rheumatoid nodules, Sjögren syndrome in up to 20%, and rarely amyloidosis.[45,46] Cricoarytenoid joints may exhibit erosion and ankylosis, resulting in restriction of joint mobility, dysphonia, stridor, globus sensation, dysphagia, odyno-phagia, and coughing. Laryngoscopy may demonstrate thickened mucosa overlying the arytenoids, glottic chink, bowing of the vocal folds, and some degree of arytenoid fixation. CT and direct laryngoscopy can be used to assess the cricoarytenoid joints. Rheumatoid nodules have been described on the true and false vocal folds and over-lying the arytenoids; they are more common in patients who test positive for rheuma-toid factor on serology. Rheumatoid nodules may resemble simple vocal fold nodules; however, histology reveals a central zone of fibrinous necrosis surrounded by fibro-blasts, histiocytes, and monocytes. Nodules tend to occur in regions of microtrauma and are often associated with edema and fibrosis. Treatment consists of systemic or intrajoint steroids and DMARDs. Large symptom-causing rheumatoid nodules may require resection; tracheostomy is indicated in cases of airway compromise.[46]

Sjögren Syndrome

Sjögren syndrome is characterized by lymphocytic infiltration of secretory glands. It affects salivary and lacrimal glands, resulting in sicca syndrome, xerostomia, throat dryness, and keratoconjunctivitis.[45,47] The effect on minor salivary glands results in mucosal dryness, dysphagia, dysphonia, and nonproductive cough.[45] Sjögren may be primary or secondary to other autoimmune disorders. Primary Sjögren can have pulmonary, renal, neurologic, cutaneous, and musculoskeletal involvement.[47] Serology positive for SS-A or SS-B autoantibodies or salivary gland biopsy can be diagnostic. Treatment includes local symptom-reducing agents such as sialogogues and saliva substitutes, steroids, and DMARDs.[47]

Systemic Lupus Erythematosus

Systemic lupus erythematosus is characterized by immune complex–mediated damage to blood vessels, mucosal and serosal surfaces, and connective tissues; it can affect most organ systems with a predilection for kidneys, joints, skin, the nervous system, and lungs. Up to one-third of patients have laryngeal involvement presenting with dysphonia, dyspnea, and occasionally dysphagia or odynopha-gia.[48,49] Laryngoscopy demonstrates edema, erythema, rheumatoid nodules, and occasionally vocal fold immobility. Subglottic stenosis has been reported. Patho-physiology of laryngeal inflammation is not well understood but could be related to deposition of immunoglobulin or immune complexes along the basement mem-brane. Vasculitis is rarely seen on laryngeal biopsy. Treatment consists of steroids and DMARDs.[49]

Mucous Membrane Pemphigoid

Mucous membrane pemphigoid (MMP) is group of chronic autoimmune subepithelial blistering diseases primarily affecting mucous membranes; circulating antibodies target various basement membrane zone antigens. MMP may present with laryngeal erosions rather than blisters, edema, synechiae, or stenosis. Symptoms include dysphonia and dyspnea. Subepithelial bullae and inflammatory cell infiltration can be seen on histology; immunofluorescence may demonstrate deposition of IgG, IgA, and/or C3 in the basement membrane zone of mucosa. MMP should be sus-pected in patients with skin or other mucous membrane lesions (especially oral or ocular). Treatment consists of dapsone and/or sulfasalazine, steroids, and DMARDs.[50]

SUMMARY

Chronic laryngitis may result from a wide variety of conditions, and its symptoms and laryngoscopy findings are often nonspecific. Chronic laryngitis may occasionally present with airway compromise requiring immediate intervention. Many causes of chronic laryngitis may mimic laryngeal carcinoma; however, concurrent carcinoma may also exist.

REFERENCES

1. Wood JM, Athanasiadis T, Allen J. Laryngitis. BMJ 2014;349:g5827. Available at: http://www.ncbi.nlm.nih.gov/pubmed/25300640. Accessed September 9, 2018.
2. Stein DJ, Noordzij JP. Incidence of chronic laryngitis. Ann Otol Rhinol Laryngol 2013;122(12):771–4.
3. Thomas CM, Jetté ME, Clary MS. Factors associated with infectious laryngitis: a retrospective review of 15 cases. Ann Otol Rhinol Laryngol 2017;126(5):388–95.
4. Carpenter PS, Kendall KA. MRSA chronic bacterial laryngitis: a growing problem. Laryngoscope 2018;128(4):921–5.
5. Kinnari TJ, Lampikoski H, Hyyrynen T, et al. Bacterial biofilm associated with chronic laryngitis. Arch Otolaryngol Head Neck Surg 2012;138(5):467.
6. Eliashar R, Gross M, Goldfarb A, et al. Purulent chondritis of the laryngeal framework cartilages. Ann Otol Rhinol Laryngol 2005;114(3):219–22.
7. Amoils CP, Shindo ML. Laryngotracheal manifestations of Rhinoscleroma. Ann Otol Rhinol Laryngol 1996;105(5):336–40.
8. El Ayoubi F, Chariba I, El Ayoubi A, et al. Primary tuberculosis of the larynx. Eur Ann Otorhinolaryngol Head Neck Dis 2014;131(6):361–4.
9. Bailey CM, Windle-Taylor PC. Tuberculous laryngitis: a series of 37 patients. Laryngoscope 1981;91(1):93–100. Available at: http://www.ncbi.nlm.nih.gov/pubmed/6779070. Accessed August 31, 2018.
10. Goughenour KD, Rappleye CA. Antifungal therapeutics for dimorphic fungal pathogens. Virulence 2017;8(2):211–21.
11. Ward PH, Morledge D, Berci G, et al. Coccidioidomycosis of the larynx in infants and adults. Ann Otol Rhinol Laryngol 1977;86(5):655–60.
12. Garcia I, Barbella R, Dickson S, et al. Paracoccidioidomycosis (South American Blastomycosis) of the larynx mimicking carcinoma. Am J Med Sci 2008;335(2):149–50.
13. Sant'Anna GD, Mauri M, Arrarte JL, et al. Laryngeal manifestations of paracoccidioidomycosis (South American blastomycosis). Arch Otolaryngol Head Neck Surg 1999;125(12):1375–8. Available at: http://www.ncbi.nlm.nih.gov/pubmed/10604418. Accessed July 19, 2018.
14. Pochini Sobrinho F, Della Negra M, Queiroz W, et al. Histoplasmosis of the larynx. Braz J Otorhinolaryngol 2007;73(6):857–61.
15. Ansari HA, Saeed N, Khan N, et al. Laryngeal histoplasmosis. BMJ Case Rep 2016;2016 [pii:bcr2016216423].
16. Rucci J, Eisinger G, Miranda-Gomez G, et al. Blastomycosis of the head and neck. Am J Otolaryngol 2014;35(3):390–5.
17. Boyle JO, Coulthard SW, Mandel RM. Laryngeal involvement in disseminated coccidioidomycosis. Arch Otolaryngol Head Neck Surg 1991;117(4):433–8. Available at: http://www.ncbi.nlm.nih.gov/pubmed/2007017. Accessed August 6, 2018.

18. Payne J, Koopmann CF. Laryngeal carcinoma–or is it laryngeal blastomycosis. Laryngoscope 1984;94(5 Pt 1):608–11. Available at: http://www.ncbi.nlm.nih. gov/pubmed/6325837. Accessed July 19, 2018.
19. Sataloff RT, Wilborn A, Prestipino A, et al. Histoplasmosis of the larynx. Am J Oto- laryngol 1993;14(3):199–205. Available at: http://www.ncbi.nlm.nih.gov/pubmed/ 8338203. Accessed August 6, 2018.
20. Tamagawa S, Hotomi M, Yuasa J, et al. Primary laryngeal cryptococcosis resem- bling laryngeal carcinoma. Auris Nasus Larynx 2015;42(4):337–40.
21. Harless L, Jiang N, Schneider F, et al. Herpes simplex virus laryngitis presenting as airway obstruction: a case report and literature review. Ann Otol Rhinol Lar- yngol 2017;126(5):424–8.
22. Hawkshaw MJ, Pebdani P, Sataloff RT. Reflux laryngitis: an update, 2009–2012. J Voice 2013;27(4):486–94.
23. Altman KW, Prufer N, Vaezi MF. A review of clinical practice guidelines for reflux disease: toward creating a clinical protocol for the otolaryngologist. Laryngo- scope 2011;121(4):717–23.
24. Asaoka D, Nagahara A, Matsumoto K, et al. Current perspectives on reflux laryn- gitis. Clin J Gastroenterol 2014;7(6):471–5.
25. Ahmed TF, Khandwala F, Abelson TI, et al. Chronic laryngitis associated with gastroesophageal reflux: prospective assessment of differences in practice pat- terns between gastroenterologists and ENT physicians. Am J Gastroenterol 2006; 101(3):470–8.
26. Simpson CB, Sulica L, Postma GN, et al. Idiopathic ulcerative laryngitis. Laryngo- scope 2011;121(5):1023–6.
27. Haft S, Farquhar D, Carey R, et al. Anticholinergic use is a major risk factor for dysphonia. Ann Otol Rhinol Laryngol 2015;124(10):797–802.
28. Woo P, Casper J, Colton R, et al. Dysphonia in the aging. Laryngoscope 1992; 102(2):139–44.
29. Dworkin JP. Laryngitis: types, causes, and treatments. Otolaryngol Clin North Am 2008;41(2):419–36.
30. Benninger MS, Murry T. The singer's voice. San Diego, CA: Plural Publishing, Inc; 2008.
31. Stachler RJ, Dworkin-Valenti JP. Allergic laryngitis. Curr Opin Otolaryngol Head Neck Surg 2017;25(3):242–6.
32. Krouse JH. Allergy and laryngeal disorders. Curr Opin Otolaryngol Head Neck Surg 2016;24(3):221–5.
33. Dean CM, Sataloff RT, Hawkshaw MJ, et al. Laryngeal sarcoidosis. J Voice 2002; 16(2):283–8. Available at: http://www.ncbi.nlm.nih.gov/pubmed/12150382. Ac- cessed July 19, 2018.
34. Sims HS, Thakkar KH. Airway involvement and obstruction from granulomas in African–American patients with sarcoidosis. Respir Med 2007;101(11):2279–83.
35. Plaschke CC, Owen HH, Rasmussen N. Clinically isolated laryngeal sarcoidosis. Eur Arch Otorhinolaryngol 2011;268(4):575–80.
36. Neel HB, McDonald TJ. Laryngeal sarcoidosis. Ann Otol Rhinol Laryngol 1982; 91(4):359–62.
37. Raymond AK, Sneige N, Batsakis JG. Amyloidosis in the upper aerodigestive tracts. Ann Otol Rhinol Laryngol 1992;101(9):794–6.
38. Phillips NM, Matthews E, Altmann C, et al. Laryngeal amyloidosis: diagnosis, pathophysiology and management. J Laryngol Otol 2017;131(S2):S41–7.
39. Pribitkin E, Friedman O, O'Hara B, et al. Amyloidosis of the upper aerodigestive tract. Laryngoscope 2003;113(12):2095–101.

40. Rudy SF, Jeffery CC, Damrose EJ. Clinical characteristics of laryngeal versus nonlaryngeal amyloidosis. Laryngoscope 2018;128(3):670–4.
41. Trimarchi M, Sinico RA, Teggi R, et al. Otorhinolaryngological manifestations in granulomatosis with polyangiitis (Wegener's). Autoimmun Rev 2013;12(4):501–5.
42. Langford CA, Sneller MC, Hallahan CW, et al. Clinical features and therapeutic management of subglottic stenosis in patients with Wegener's granulomatosis. Arthritis Rheum 1996;39(10):1754–60. Available at: http://www.ncbi.nlm.nih.gov/pubmed/8843868. Accessed September 9, 2018.
43. Mathian A, Miyara M, Cohen-Aubart F, et al. Relapsing polychondritis: a 2016 update on clinical features, diagnostic tools, treatment and biological drug use. Best Pract Res Clin Rheumatol 2016;30(2):316–33.
44. Tasli H, Birkent H, Gerek M. Three cases of relapsing polycondritis with isolated laryngotracheal stenosis. Turk Arch Otorhinolaryngol 2017;55(2):77–82.
45. Brooker DS. Rheumatoid arthritis: otorhinolaryngological manifestations. Clin Otolaryngol Allied Sci 1988;13(3):239–46. Available at: http://www.ncbi.nlm.nih.gov/pubmed/3042209. Accessed July 20, 2018.
46. Voulgari PV, Papazisi D, Bai M, et al. Laryngeal involvement in rheumatoid arthritis. Rheumatol Int 2005;25(5):321–5.
47. Both T, Dalm VASH, van Hagen PM, et al. Reviewing primary Sjögren's syndrome: beyond the dryness - From pathophysiology to diagnosis and treatment. Int J Med Sci 2017;14(3):191–200.
48. Woo P, Mendelsohn J, Humphrey D. Rheumatoid nodules of the larynx. Otolaryngol Head Neck Surg 1995;113(1):147–50.
49. Teitel AD, MacKenzie CR, Stern R, et al. Laryngeal involvement in systemic lupus erythematosus. Semin Arthritis Rheum 1992;22(3):203–14. Available at: http://www.ncbi.nlm.nih.gov/pubmed/1295093. Accessed September 10, 2018.
50. Alexandre M, Brette M-D, Pascal F, et al. A prospective study of upper aerodigestive tract manifestations of mucous membrane pemphigoid. Medicine (Baltimore) 2006;85(4):239–52.

Presbyphonia and Minimal Glottic Insufficiency

David E. Rosow, MD*, Debbie R. Pan, BA

KEYWORDS

- Presbyphonia • Glottic insufficiency • Voice disorder • Elderly • Aging voice
- Quality of life

KEY POINTS

- Presbyphonia is becoming more prevalent as both a quality-of-life concern and a treatable medical condition as the elderly population continues to grow in the United States.
- Many age-related physiologic changes contribute to the clinical symptoms of presbyphonia, such as deterioration of voice quality and vocal strain.
- Diagnostic evaluation of presbyphonia relies on stroboscopy as the gold standard to assess glottic insufficiency.
- Many interventions, including voice therapy, vocal fold injection augmentation, or thyroplasty, can be of benefit to patients seeking voice improvement.

INTRODUCTION

According to the US Department of Health and Human Services, the elderly population aged 65 years or older numbered approximately 49.2 million in 2016, the most recent year data were available, representing an increase of 33% since 2006. It is estimated that now approximately 1 in every 7 Americans is elderly.[1] This finding is paralleled by a similar increase projected by the United Nations Report on Ageing, which predicted that between 2015 and 2030, the number of people in the world older than 60 years old would grow by 56%, from 901 million to 1.4 billion, and that by 2050, the global population of this age would reach nearly 2.1 billion.[2] As the population of older people continues to increase, there has been a reported parallel increase in the number of elderly patients seeking medical attention due to voice concerns.[3] Presbyphonia, or aging of the voice, is a clinical diagnosis given to patients who experience a constellation of vocal symptoms due to natural anatomic and physiologic changes that come with age. Common symptoms include increased vocal effort leading to deterioration of

Disclosure Statement: The authors have nothing to disclose.
Department of Otolaryngology, University of Miami Miller School of Medicine, 1120 Northwest 14th Street, 5th Floor, Miami, FL 33136, USA
* Corresponding author.
E-mail address: drosow@med.miami.edu

voice quality, altered pitch, reduction in volume, vocal roughness, breathiness, and vocal fatigue; however, elderly patients most commonly present to an otolaryngologist with a complaint as simple as self-reported "hoarseness."[4,5]

Although it is debated whether presbyphonia should even be considered a pathologic condition given its organic nature, there is clear consensus about its negative effect on quality of life for the individuals affected. Patients report experiencing increased anxiety and frustration over their voice quality, and in particular, the consequent necessity to repeat oneself in conversation. Some avoid social situations because of this frustration, leading to decreased quality of life.[4,6] In addition, one must acknowledge the plethora of other age-related conditions or circumstances that may affect communication for the elderly and further reduce quality of life. One study found that elderly individuals with hearing loss were more than twice as likely to have coexisting dysphonia than those without hearing loss and that these individuals with concurrent impairments had greater depression scores compared with those with neither.[7] Voice problems can also influence a listener's perspective of the elderly speaker and negatively impact interpersonal relationships over time. It is with these considerations in mind that the authors aim to help the reader learn more about how to identify and treat presbyphonia to significantly improve the aging experience for elderly patients. This article focuses on recent advancements guiding current understanding of the pathophysiology, acoustic and clinical symptoms, diagnosis, and treatment of presbyphonia.

EPIDEMIOLOGY OF THE AGING VOICE

Although the exact prevalence is unknown, presbyphonia is one of the primary reasons for voice concern visits among the treatment-seeking elderly population.[3] Several studies have estimated that voice disorders affect up to 30% of individuals aged 60 years or older.[4,8] Despite these estimates, presbyphonia is likely underreported due to patient perception of the condition. In a cross-sectional study, nearly 25% of surveyed elderly individuals with dysphonia thought that their voice disorder was a normal part of aging, and as many as 50% were unaware that treatments were available.[9] To some degree, presbyphonia is simply an aftereffect of normal physiologic changes to laryngeal structure and organization; however, it is important to note that a definable condition resulting from physiologic change does not preclude it from having identifiable risk factors and proven treatment measures, just as with a pathologic process. Significant reported risk factors for symptoms of presbyphonia include esophageal reflux, chronic pain or chronic disease, and vocal abuse.[3,4] The presence of these comorbidities may negatively impact an elderly patient's ability to compensate for the physiologic changes that occur to the vocal folds with aging. Reducing these exposures as well as increasing an elderly individual's awareness of proper management of dysphonia will thus certainly improve the overall health of this population group.

THEORIES ON PATHOPHYSIOLOGY

Presbyphonia is driven by numerous anatomic and physiologic changes involved in the aging of the voice. Although many studies have been conducted to elucidate the pathophysiology behind presbyphonia, it is most accurate to say there are contributions from a variety of processes, such as age-related changes in the laryngeal musculature, adjacent soft tissue, mucosa, and cartilage. Perhaps the most prominent theory is one of muscle atrophy. Several studies support the idea that there is a weakening or loss of contractile elements and forces within the thyroarytenoid muscle as aging occurs. Martins and colleagues[10] conducted morphometric analyses of 200 muscle fibers per vocal fold in 30 cadavers, with data collected equally among 3 age groups: ages 30 to 50 years as control, 60 to 75 years, and 76 to 90 years. The mean diameter of vocal muscle fibers in the elderly age groups was smaller than in the control ($P<.01$), with the smallest diameter reported in the oldest age group. However, more recently published literature has contributed findings that challenge the role of thyroarytenoid muscle atrophy in presbyphonia. Two independent studies investigated thyroarytenoid muscle volume via MRI, comparing size differences across different age groups, and both found that there was no statistically significant volumetric change in the thyroarytenoid muscle with aging.[11,12]

Other theories include age-related calcification of supporting hyaline cartilages as well as decreased neuromuscular control via decreased density of nerve fibers within the larynx over time.[13–15] Connor and colleagues[14] investigated the neuromuscular junctions of the thyroarytenoid muscle in a rat model and discovered that there were significant changes with aging that were comparable to what was observed in denervated muscle. These findings were supported by another study that found that aging was associated with a reduction of both sensory and secretomotor nerve endings in the F344/N rat larynx.[15]

From a cellular perspective, there are changes at the microstructural level of the larynx to consider in presbyphonia. The vocal folds are composed of 5 histologically distinct layers: epithelium, superficial lamina propria, intermediate lamina propria, deep lamina propria, and the vocalis bundle of the thyroarytenoid muscle. The superficial lamina propria has low levels of collagen and elastin; the intermediate layer has some collagen and higher levels of elastin, and the deep layer contains abundant levels of fibrous proteins, such as collagen with lower levels of elastin.[16] In a general sense, the elastic fibers are located more principally in the outer layers of the vocal fold, whereas the collagen fibers are predominantly in the deep layers; this organization allows for the vocal folds to have vibratory capability from its more superficial layers while being steadily anchored by deeper layers.[17] The normal extracellular matrix distributed across the 3 layers are interweaved and confer the ability of the vocal folds to be stretched during phonation.[5]

With aging, the most widely described changes occur within the lamina propria. There are multiple studies that discuss an age-related increase in collagen as well as decrease in elastic fibers and hyaluronic acid within the superficial lamina propria. These changes cause stiffness that compromises the viscoelastic properties of the vocal folds and manifests as dysphonia in the elderly. Collagenase enzymatic expression has been found to be suppressed in elderly vocal folds, which may explain the increased collagen levels described in this age group.[18] Other histologic changes in the connective tissue matrix have been noted with aging, including an increased relative number of type I collagen fibers, disorganized collagen bundle formation and distribution, and reduced elastic fiber density due to less active fibroblastic activity.[19,20] Hyaluronic acid also plays a role in the viscoelasticity of the vocal folds by providing pliability and impact absorption properties. According to a study that analyzed hyaluronic acid levels from cadaveric vocal folds via immunohistochemistry, hyaluronic acid levels in the lamina propria reduced by almost 50% for men older than 60 years old.[21] The wide array of physiologic changes (as well as examples of conflicting findings) described in the aging larynx, from both structural and functional standpoints, reveals that the pathophysiology behind presbyphonia is likely a more complex concept than previously thought.

CLINICAL AND ACOUSTIC MANIFESTATIONS

Several clinical signs and acoustic alterations affecting the human voice have been thoroughly described as consequences of aging. Along with declining pulmonary function, the older adult experiences acoustic shifts impacting voice quality, including decreased volume and vocal intensity, narrowed register, decreased maximum duration of phonation, instability in fundamental frequency, increased jitter and shimmer, and increased breathiness.[16,22,23] These measures allow the physician to clinically infer instability of vocal mechanics, such as insufficient glottic closure or abnormal vocal fold vibratory movements. Jitter and shimmer in particular have been found to independently contribute to a perceived aged quality of the voice.[24] However, the elderly population is a heterogeneous group, and the presentation of presbyphonia may be variable among individuals.

In fact, even between genders, there have been key differences reported in the pattern with which the voice changes with aging. For example, acoustic analyses have demonstrated that the mean fundamental frequency in women decreases over time, whereas in men, the mean fundamental frequency decreases until they reach their mid- to late 40s, after which an increase is noted as they continue to age.[16,23] According to Awan,[25] the most prominent feature of presbyphonia in women is the observed decrease in mean fundamental frequency of their speaking voice. Regarding breathy voice quality, it has been reported that age-related increases in breathiness are more pronounced in men compared with women, although both older groups trend similarly when compared with their younger counterparts.[26] These age-related alterations can be quite noticeable and possibly alarming to the individual or to those with whom the individual interacts. It is important that the physician be aware of these clinical manifestations when performing a thorough assessment of a patient with suspected presbyphonia.

DIAGNOSTIC EVALUATION

An accurate evaluation of presbyphonia begins with keeping in mind aspects of the patient's voice that would reflect anticipated acoustic changes as mentioned above. An assessment should include a thorough and focused history and physical examination. Suggestions for pertinent questions to consider are listed in **Table 1**. However, although history and physical examinations are important, it has been reported that when these assessments are done without stroboscopy to evaluate dysphonia, they have a diagnostic accuracy as low as 5%.[27] Stroboscopy has become the primary method for diagnosing presbyphonia because of its ease of use and reliability.

Table 1
Key vocal features to note during history-taking in the elderly

Vocal Features	Focused History
Difficulty projecting	Do you have difficulty being heard over background noise?
Increased breathiness	Do you feel like you are losing air or sighing when you talk?
Decreased volume	Do others ask you to repeat yourself more frequently than in the past?
Vocal fatigue	Has it gotten harder to keep up with your day-to-day vocal demands?
Narrowed register	Does your voice break/crack in conversation or while singing?
Unstable/altered F_0	Men: Has your voice gotten noticeably higher over time? Women: Has your voice gotten noticeably lower over time?

Hallmark laryngeal findings for dysphonia in the elderly (noted in **Fig. 1**) include bowing of the vocal fold margin or increased concavity of the vocal folds, prominent vocal processes of the arytenoid cartilage, and notable glottic insufficiency during phonation.[5,16,23] Furthermore, the viscoelastic properties of the superficial lamina propria can be examined with this method to reveal asymmetry or changes in the mucosal wave; these observations would not be possible to note with conventional laryngoscopy. In patients with presbyphonia, the stroboscopic light source may experience difficulty syncing with the unstable frequency and unsustained phonation produced by the vocal folds; thus, images of the vibratory cycle can be blurry and may not resemble the clear, crisp images expected from a normal stroboscopic examination.[16] One recent study found that using continuous light endoscopy to visualize vocal fold bowing during phonation had a 93.6% diagnostic sensitivity compared with stroboscopy, and the s/z ratio (the ratio of time a patient can sustain the "s" and "z" sounds, used as an indicator of laryngeal pathologic condition) had a specificity of 91.4%, suggesting their respective utilities as initial diagnostic tests for glottic insufficiency in presbyphonia if necessary.[28] Despite these findings, the investigators of the study still affirmed the use of stroboscopy as the best method of diagnostic evaluation for presbyphonia.

When considering a diagnosis of presbyphonia in an elderly patient, it is important to keep in mind that there may be concurrent organic disease primarily responsible for the voice disorder. In patients over the age of 60 years, benign vocal fold lesions, such as polyps and nodules, are the most common causes of hoarseness, with malignant lesions and vocal fold paralysis recognized as other common causes.[5] Elderly patients can also have concurrent neurologic disorders, such as Parkinson disease, or chronic inflammatory conditions that can cause glottic insufficiency.[23] When evaluating an elderly patient with dysphonia, it becomes crucial to rule out these diseases or any other suspected cause by history, physical examination, and appropriate testing first before committing to presbyphonia as a diagnosis of exclusion.

CURRENT TREATMENT OPTIONS

An early, accurate identification of presbyphonia allows for the possibility of prompt treatment and even possible restoration of the voice. There are many effective options that are currently available and being used for these patients, including voice therapy,

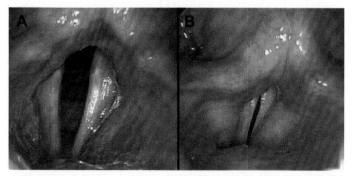

Fig. 1. (A) Stroboscopic images from a 75-year-old man with presbyphonia. Bowing and concavity of the vocal folds is noted on abduction (B), with glottic insufficiency noted during phonation.

injection augmentation, and medialization thyroplasty surgery. Regrettably, 2 recent studies have shown that a very low percentage of elderly adults seek treatment for voice disorders, 10% and 14.6%, respectively.[4,29] This low rate is especially unfortunate, because these studies also found that up to 50% of these patients who sought treatment saw voice improvement. These findings suggest that more effort needs to be placed in making older adults with dysphonia aware of the availability and efficacy of treatment.

Voice therapy is one of the mainstays of treatment of presbyphonia and many other voice disorders. It focuses on improving the quality of the voice by incorporating phonatory exercises to address concerns of respiratory support, voice hygiene, vocal-related quality of life, and optimal laryngeal function.[30,31] One recently published study showed that intensive voice therapy (4 times per week) reduced the degree of observed vocal fold bowing by more than 38% compared with a group receiving therapy twice per week.[32] Voice therapy is therefore an intervention that has been proven beneficial to patients and is usually offered first due to its noninvasive nature.

Injection augmentation is another treatment option that is commonly used in the treatment of presbyphonia, with materials such as fat, hyaluronic acid, carboxymethylcellulose, and calcium hydroxylapatite injected into the vocal folds to restore glottic competence.[31] When selecting the material for injection, several factors should be considered, including reabsorption of the material by the body, anticipated inflammatory response, and desired timing between injections.[33] Injections are performed deep in the paraglottic space, because there is so far no available material that matches the viscoelastic properties of human superficial lamina propria.[34] The viscosity of the substance should be accounted for, because stiffer materials, such as calcium hydroxylapatite, may restrict the vibration of the superficial lamina propria when injected deep to this layer. In contrast, low viscosity substances, such as carboxymethylcellulose or hyaluronic acid, are more pliable, easier to inject, and do not restrict vibration of the lamina propria, but they do not last as long and are theoretically more likely to run the risk of spreading along unanticipated anatomic planes after injection.[33,35] However, there is evidence that hyaluronic acid injections can be reversed if there are complications due to the availability of injectable hyaluronidase, an additional benefit when compared with other injectable materials.[36] It has also been shown that hyaluronic acid injections may even promote tissue regeneration, contributing to the recruitment of fibroblasts and increased transcription of collagen, as supported by an in vivo study in a rabbit model.[37] Finally, injection augmentation can be done in a minimally invasive fashion in an office setting with local anesthesia only, which is often ideal for elderly patients who may have hesitations or medical comorbidities preventing procedures in an operating room under sedation or general anesthesia.

If warranted, surgical techniques are available and effective, with medialization thyroplasty recognized as the standard. Although this surgery cannot correct the muscular or the properties of the lamina propria associated with presbyphonia, it provides a correction of the shape of the vocal fold (**Fig. 2**) to reduce glottic insufficiency.[38] Research on the impact of thyroplasty on patients with presbyphonia has shown increased ease of phonation as well as improvement in voice quality and voice-related quality of life.[38,39] Although the specifics of the surgical procedure are not discussed here, it should be noted that the procedure is usually completed under local anesthesia with minimal sedation, making it more suitable for elderly patients with comorbid conditions than other procedures that might require general anesthesia.

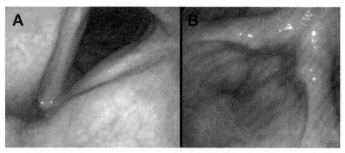

Fig. 2. (A) Stroboscopic images from the same 75-year-old man with presbyphonia, taken 8 months after bilateral medialization thyroplasty. The vocal folds have a markedly more convex appearance during abduction (B), with complete glottic closure noted during phonation.

As medicine becomes more technologically advanced, future direction for presbyphonia treatment may involve reversal of the underlying mechanisms responsible for age-related changes instead of the currently available repletion techniques. Targeting the physiologic changes at a cellular or molecular level allows for new approaches for treatment involving tissue engineering, lamina propria restoration, or stimulation of laryngeal factors responsible for viscoelasticity of the vocal folds. Several recent clinical trials have investigated the effects of basic fibroblast growth factor (bFGF) therapy on age-related vocal fold atrophy in humans after demonstrated increases of hyaluronic acid in rat models with bFGF injections.[40,41] Preliminary results up to 6 months after bFGF injection boast increases in Voice Handicap Index-10 scores, enhancement in voice quality according to the GRBAS (grade, roughness, breathiness, asthenia, strain) scale, increases in maximum phonation time, and improvements in other vocal acoustic measures.[41] The therapeutic benefit of treatment, whether in the form of currently existing therapies or those that are in development, tremendously aid in the restoration of voice and hope for elderly patients suffering from dysphonia.

SUMMARY

Presbyphonia is becoming increasingly prominent as the demographic worldwide continues to shift toward the geriatric population. Although the cause is complex, several physiologic explanations have been postulated to be responsible for age-related dysphonia, including changes to the musculature, surrounding cartilage, and lamina propria of the vocal folds. Presbyphonia is a diagnosis of exclusion and is diagnosed by stroboscopy revealing characteristic glottic insufficiency, with findings supported by thorough history and physical examinations. Patients often present with noticeably reduced voice quality, breathiness, hoarseness, unsteady fundamental frequency, and vocal fatigue. Often, these older individuals develop social anxiety and decreased quality of life due to poor social interactions and difficulty with communication. Many studies have demonstrated the value of treatments such as vocal therapy, injection augmentation, and medialization thyroplasty; having effective treatments offers an assurance that presbyphonia can ultimately be corrected. By instilling a greater sense of the availability, accessibility, and efficacy of treatment for those presenting with dysphonia, physicians can play crucial roles in promoting a more rewarding aging experience for their patients.

REFERENCES

1. U.S. Department of Health and Human Services. Administration on aging. Administration for community living. A profile of older Americans 2017. Available at: https://www.acl.gov/sites/default/files/Aging%20and%20Disability%20in%20America/2017OlderAmericansProfile.pdf. Accessed July 17, 2018.

2. United Nations, Department of Economic, Social Affairs, Population Division. World population ageing 2015 (ST/ESA/SER.A/390) 2015. Available at: http://www.un.org/en/development/desa/population/publications/pdf/ageing/WPA2015_Report.pdf. Accessed September 9, 2018.

3. Yamauchi A, Imagawa H, Sakakaibara K, et al. Vocal fold atrophy in a Japanese tertiary medical institute: status quo of the most aged country. J Voice 2014;28:231–6.

4. Roy N, Stemple J, Merrill RM, et al. Epidemiology of voice disorders in the elderly: preliminary findings. Laryngoscope 2007;117:628–33.

5. Kendall K. Presbyphonia: a review. Curr Opin Otolaryngol Head Neck Surg 2007;15:137–40.

6. Verdonck-de Leeuw IM, Mahieu HF. Vocal aging and the impact on daily life: a longitudinal study. J Voice 2004;18:193–202.

7. Cohen SM, Turley R. Coprevalence and impact of dysphonia and hearing loss in the elderly. Laryngoscope 2009;119:1870–3.

8. De Araújo Pernambuco L, Espelt A, Balata PM, et al. Prevalence of voice disorders in the elderly: a systematic review of population-based studies. Eur Arch Otorhinolaryngol 2015;272:2601.

9. Turley R, Cohen S. Impact of voice and swallowing problems in the elderly. Otolaryngol Head Neck Surg 2009;140(1):33–6.

10. Martins RH, Pessin AB, Nassib DJ, et al. Aging voice and the laryngeal muscle atrophy. Laryngoscope 2015;125:2518–21.

11. Ziade G, Semaan S, Ghulmiyyah J, et al. Structural and anatomic laryngeal measurements in geriatric populations using MRI. J Voice 2017;31:359–62.

12. Saint-Victor S, Barbarite E, Sidani C, et al. Volumetric analysis of vocal fold atrophy via magnetic resonance imaging. J Laryngol Otol 2018;132(9):822–6.

13. Malinowski A. Shape, dimensions and process of calcification of the cartilaginous framework of the larynx in relation to age and sex in the Polish population. Folia Morphol (Warsz) 1967;26:118–28.

14. Connor NP, Suzuki T, Lee K, et al. Neuromuscular junction changes in aged rat thyroarytenoid muscle. Ann Otol Rhinol Laryngol 2002;111(7 Pt 1):579–86.

15. Yamamoto Y, Tanaka S, Tsubone H, et al. Age-related changes in sensory and secretomotor nerve endings in the larynx of F344/N rat. Arch Gerontol Geriatr 2003;36(2):173–83.

16. Rapoport SK, Meiner J, Grant N. Voice changes in the elderly. Otolaryngol Clin North Am 2018;51(4):759–68.

17. Roberts T, Morton R, Ali-Ali S. Microstructure of the vocal fold in elderly humans. Clin Anat 2011;24:544–51.

18. Chen X, Thibeault SL. Characteristics of age-related changes in cultured human vocal fold fibroblasts. Laryngoscope 2008;118:1700–4.

19. Sato K, Hirano M, Nakashima T. Age-related changes of collagenous fibers in the human vocal fold mucosa. Ann Otol Rhinol Laryngol 2002;111:15–20.

20. Hirano M, Sato K, Nakashima T. Fibroblasts in geriatric vocal fold mucosa. Acta Otolaryngol 2000;120(2):336–40.

21. Branco A, Rodrigues SA, Fabro AT, et al. Hyaluronic acid behavior in the lamina propria of the larynx with advancing age. Otolaryngol Head Neck Surg 2014;151: 652–6.
22. Bradley JP, Johns MM III. The aging voice. In: Sataloff RT, Benninger MS, editors. Sataloff's comprehensive textbook of otolaryngology head and neck surgery: laryngology. New Delhi (India): JP Medical Publishers Ltd; 2015. p. 635–40.
23. Kost KM, Sataloff RT. Voice disorders in the elderly. Clin Geriatr Med 2018;34(2): 191–203.
24. Gregory ND, Chandran S, Lurie D, et al. Voice disorders in the elderly. J Voice 2012;26:254–8.
25. Awan SN. The aging female voice: acoustic and respiratory data. Clin Linguist Phon 2006;20:171–80.
26. Linville SE. Source characteristics of aged voice assessed from long-term average spectra. J Voice 2002;16:472–9.
27. Myint C, Moore JE, Hu A, et al. A comparison of initial and subsequent follow-up strobovideolaryngoscopic examinations in singers. J Voice 2016;30(4):472–7.
28. Vaca M, Cobeta I, Mora E, et al. Clinical assessment of glottic insufficiency in age-related dysphonia. J Voice 2017;31(1):128.e1–5.
29. Bertelsen C, Zhou S, Hapner ER, et al. Socioeconomic characteristics and treatment response among aging adults with voice disorders in the United States. JAMA Otolaryngol Head Neck Surg 2018;144(8):719–26.
30. Ford C. Voice restoration in presbyphonia. Arch Otolaryngol Head Neck Surg 2004;130:1117.
31. Bradley JP, Hapner E, Johns MM III. What is the optimal treatment for presbyphonia? Laryngoscope 2014;124(11):2439–40.
32. Godoy J, Silverio K, Brasolotto A. Effectiveness of vocal therapy for the elderly when applying conventional and intensive approaches: a randomized clinical trial. J Voice 2018. https://doi.org/10.1016/j.jvoice.2018.03.017.
33. Lisi C, Hawkshaw MJ, Sataloff RT. Viscosity of materials for laryngeal injection: a review of current knowledge and clinical implications. J Voice 2012;27:119–23.
34. Caton T, Thibeault SL, Klemuk S, et al. Viscoelasticity of hyaluronan and nonhyaluronan based vocal fold injectables: implications for mucosal versus muscle use. Laryngoscope 2007;117:516–21.
35. Remacle M, Lawson G. Injectable substances or vocal fold augmentation. Otolaryngol Head Neck Surg 2001;9:393–7.
36. Woo P. Hyaluronidase injection in the vocal folds for vocal hemorrhage, Reinke edema, and hyaluronic acid overinjection: a novel application in the larynx. J Voice 2018;32(4):492–8.
37. Thibeault SL, Klemuk SA, Chen X, et al. In vivo engineering of the vocal fold ECM with injectable HA hydrogels—late effects on tissue repair and biomechanics in a rabbit model. J Voice 2011;25:249–53.
38. Isshiki N, Kojima H, Shoji K, et al. Vocal fold atrophy and its surgical treatment. Ann Otol Rhinol Laryngol 1996;105:182–8.
39. Postma GN, Blalock PD, Koufman JA. Bilateral medialization laryngoplasty. Laryngoscope 1998;108:1429–34.
40. Hirano S, Tateya I, Kishimoto Y, et al. Clinical trial of regeneration of aged vocal folds with growth factor therapy. Laryngoscope 2012;122:327–31.
41. Ohno S, Hirano S, Yasumoto A, et al. Outcome of regenerative therapy for age-related vocal fold atrophy with basic fibroblast growth factor. Laryngoscope 2016;126:1844–8.

Reinke's Edema

Raluca Tavaluc, MD[a], Melin Tan-Geller, MD[b,c],*

KEYWORDS

- Reinke's edema • Reinke's space • Dyspnea • Smoking cessation • Dysplasia
- Microflap techiniques

KEY POINTS

- Reinke's edema is a benign polypoid degeneration of one or both vocal folds.
- Women present most frequently with dysphonia.
- Risk factors include cigarette smoke, voice abuse, and reflux control, and increase post-intervention recurrence if not controlled.
- Dysphonia is improved but rarely resolved after intervention.
- Surgical resection with microflap techniques is mainstay, although office-based use of lasers has recently been investigated.

INTRODUCTION

Reinke's edema (RE) is a benign disease of the vocal folds. It is also referred to as polypoid corditis, polypoid laryngitis, polypoid degeneration, and chronic hypertrophic laryngitis.[1] RE is diffuse polypoid degeneration of the entire length of one or, more commonly, both vocal folds (**Fig. 1**).

HISTORY

The typical vocal fold edema seen in RE was first described by Hajek in 1891.[2] The space that holds this edema is called Reinke's space. Friedrich Berthold Reinke defined it in a series of 2 papers, in 1895[3] and 1897.[4] In Reinke's experiments, fluid was infused in the subepithelial compartment of the vocal fold. The fluid remained bound within the space that now holds his name, Reinke's space. Reinke's space is defined as the potential space between the superficial lamina propria (SLP) and the vocal ligament.[5] The boundaries of Reinke's space are the SLP superficially, the vocal fold ligament deep, the superior and inferior arcuate line cranially and caudally, Broyle ligament anteriorly, and the arytenoid posteriorly.[6] In the twentieth century RE was officially defined as edema of Reinke's space[6] (**Table 1**).

---

[a] Department of Head and Neck Surgery, University of California Los Angeles, 200 Medical Plaza, Suite 550, Los Angeles, CA 90025, USA; [b] ENT&Allergy Associates, 222 Bloomingdale Road, Suite 205, White Plains, NY 10506, USA; [c] Department of Otolaryngology, Albert Einstein College of Medicine, 1300 Morris Park Avenue, Bronx, NY 10461, USA
* Corresponding author. ENT&Allergy Associates, 222 Bloomingdale Road, Suite 205, White Plains, NY 10506, USA
E-mail address: melintangeller@gmail.com

Otolaryngol Clin N Am 52 (2019) 627–635
https://doi.org/10.1016/j.otc.2019.03.006
0030-6665/19/© 2019 Elsevier Inc. All rights reserved.

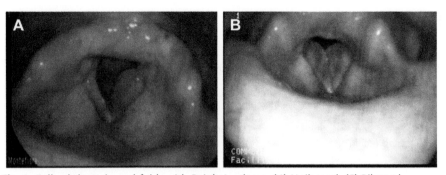

Fig. 1. Fully abducted vocal folds with Reinke's edema. (*A*) Unilateral. (*B*) Bilateral.

DEMOGRAPHICS

RE prevalence in the general population is reported to be less than 1%.[7] No epidemiologic studies report incidence based on ethnicity or geographic location. Looking at all comers undergoing suspension microlaryngoscopic procedures, RE rate has been reported at 16%.[8] Most studies report a higher incidence in women, although a few authors have found a predilection in males.[7,9]

CLINICAL PRESENTATION

The clinical presentation is dependent on the size of the lesion. In a majority of the cases, the lesions are bilateral, although usually asymmetric.[9] Because of the load effect of the edema on the mucosal folds, the most common chief complaint is dysphonia.[7] The change in fundamental frequency (F0) is what drives the majority of chief complaints. The average female F0 is 180 to 230 Hz.[10] When afflicted by RE, F0 in women is <130 Hz and in men is <100 Hz.[10] It is proposed that females seek treatment more frequently, as the decrease in F0, and the shift from female to male range is more audibly apparent (**Fig. 2**).

Patients can also present with dyspnea, although less frequently. RE is confined to the membranous vocal fold, thus impacting voice more frequently than breathing, which is more dependent on the posterior cartilaginous vocal fold. Larger lesions, however, can present with airway obstruction, especially if other vocal fold pathology is present, such as vocal fold motion impairment.[10]

During office evaluation, stroboscopic findings range based on the altered viscoelastic properties of the SLP. Most frequently, there is an enlargement of Reinke's space with associated increase of mucosal wave, increased amplitude, and asymmetry. To fully assess the size of the lesion, the forced inspiration maneuver is crucial.[11]

| Table 1 | |
Reinke's space boundaries	
Superficial	Superficial lamina propria
Deep	Vocal fold ligament
Cranial	Superior arcuate line
Caudal	Inferior arcuate line
Anterior	Broyle ligament
Posterior	Arytenoid

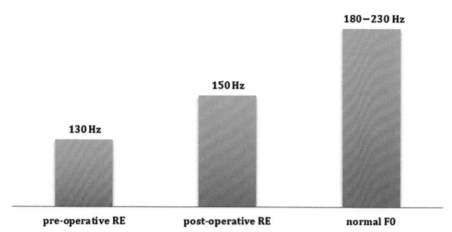

Fig. 2. Average fundamental frequency (F0) in women in RE preoperatively and postoperatively compared with average fundamental frequency in women without RE.

Aerodynamic evaluation reveal abnormally high average subglottal pressures.[12] RE size can be graded based on percent of glottic airway obstruction due to edema[13] (**Fig. 3, Table 2**).

PATHOPHYSIOLOGY

Reinke's space is filled with loose connective tissue sheets that run in parallel with the vocal fold edges.[14] In RE, increased subepithelial vascularization develops, producing dilation of the vessels, thinning of the endothelium, and increased fenestrae, causing increased vascular permeability[15,16] (**Fig. 4**). This leads to plasma exudation and the development hollow spaces, termed neobursae, on light microscopy, and loosening of intercellular junctions on electron microscopy.[17,18]

The structural components also change. There are architectural changes in the collagen and elastin fibers that form the fibrous scaffolding of the lamina propria. In normal subjects, collagen fibers are arranged in a wicker-basket configuration. In RE, collagen fibers become interwoven and fragmented.[19] Similarly, in normal specimens, elastin fibers are arranged in thin undulated parallel lines to the epithelial basement membrane. In RE, elastin fibers gain a tangled scattered distribution.[20] Lastly, fibronectin, a structural glycoprotein precursor for collagen deposition and scar formation, is decreased in RE, leading to the theory that its absence leads to the deformability of the vocal fold characteristic of RE.[21]

RISK FACTORS

RE develops from chronic damage to the vocal folds leading to the pathophysiologic changes described previously. The most important risk factor is cigarette smoke.[22–25] Voice abuse[22] and laryngopharyngeal reflux[23,26] are also associated with an increased risk of RE. Thyroid function has been investigated without an association between hypothyroidism and RE.[27–29] Older age has been investigated with adults greater than 60 who present with dysphonia, although incidence of RE was less than 1%.[30] Research on hormone association due to female predisposition is inconclusive. No association was found with hormone replacement therapy,[27] nor sex hormone receptors found on RE specimens.[31] However, sex hormone level of testosterone and progesterone in the

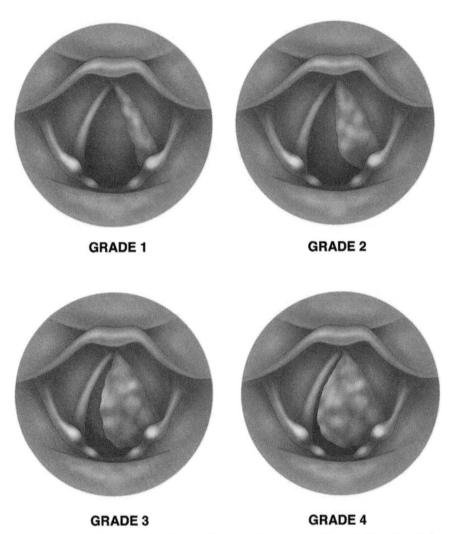

GRADE 1   **GRADE 2**

GRADE 3   **GRADE 4**

Fig. 3. Schematic drawing of Reinke's edema grading system. Illustrated by Kate Hohn. (Reprinted with permission from Tan M, Bryson PC, Pitts C, Woo P, Benninger MS. Clinical grading of Reinke's edema. The Laryngoscope 2017;127(10):2310–2313.)

body were higher, although not their ratio.[32] Lastly, atopy as determined by positive skin allergy testing had no association with RE.[33]

MALIGNANCY RISK

Because cigarette smoke is a risk factor for squamous cell carcinoma and RE, the link between RE and malignancy risk has been investigated in depth.[23,34] Most lesions are seen to have no malignant potential. The incidence of dysplasia in RE ranges between 0% and 3%.[9,23,34–37] Incidence of SCC is no greater than 0.01% to 0.02%.[34–36] Marcotullio and colleagues[23] found a correlation between more severe lesion histology and daily number of cigarettes consumed and duration of exposure to cigarette smoke. The authors' recent investigation revealed no correlation

Table 2	
Reinke's edema grading definition	
	Reinke's Edema Grade
Grade 1	Minimal polypoid degeneration of the vocal fold 25% of the glottic airway
Grade 2	Expanded polypoid lesion 25% to 50% of the glottic airway
Grade 3	Expanded polypoid lesion 50% to 75% of the glottic airway
Grade 4	Obstructive lesion regardless of laterality beyond 75% of the glottic airway

between severity of dysplasia, pack year smoking history, and size of RE lesion (unpublished results, Tan-Geller, 2018; **Table 3**).

Some authors hypothesized that RE is actually a protective pathology. Using microarray analysis, RE vocal folds have increased antioxidant gene expression.[38] Experiments with cigarette smoke extracts also showed a chemoprotective mechanism pathway inducing autophagy and antioxidant response in vitro.[39,40]

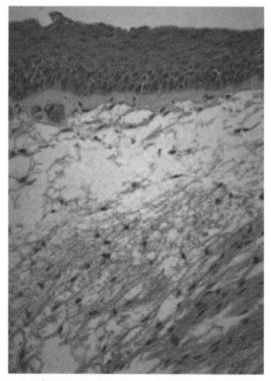

Fig. 4. Histologic image of Reinke's edema. Note the lack of cellularity and the presence of epithelial basement membrane thickening, edematous lakes, extravascular erythrocytes, and increased thickness of submucosal vessels. (Reprinted with permission from Hantzakos A, Remacle M, Dikkers FG, et al. Exudative lesions of Reinke's space: a terminology proposal. Eur Arch Otorhinolaryngol 2009;266(6):869–878.)

Table 3	
Reinke's Edema risk factors investigated	
Strong Evidence	**Weak or no Evidence**
Cigarette smoke	Hypothyroidism
Voice abuse	Older age
Laryngopharyngeal reflux	Allergic atopy
	Hormone replacement therapy

TREATMENT

The goal of treatment is symptomatic improvement of dysphonia with a primary emphasis on removal of etiologic factors. The initial treatment strategy is to remove all predisposing risk factors. Therefore, patients should be counseled on smoking cessation, undergo voice therapy, and, if applicable, control gastroesophageal reflux as initial steps.[12,41] Prior investigations on the effect of complete smoking cessation as the only treatment revealed that it did not cause reversal, but did halt the progression and, in some, helped decrease the lesion size and improve voice, although none normalized.[42]

Medical treatment options investigated are limited to steroids. Inhaled steroids have been tried in a double-blinded randomized control trial with beclomethasone dipropionate, which did not show any effect after 1 month of treatment.[43] Tateya and colleagues[44] reported the use of triamcinolone acetonide injection into Reinke's space in what the group defined mild RE with improvement in both objective and subjective voice.

In more severe cases, where either the voice handicap is high for the patient and conservative measures have yielded limited improvement in dysphonia, or when lesions cause symptomatic dyspnea, surgery is indicated. Surgically, the principle is to provide a balance of polypoid resection to decrease the redundant mucosa yet not result in a postoperative stiff vocal fold and a worsened voice. The initial surgical therapy adopted was suspension microdirect laryngoscopy with stripping of the vocal folds and decortication. This technique, however, resulted in prolonged aphonia and increased risk of anterior glottic web formation.[45] Now microflap techniques with careful reduction of the gelatinous matrix, redraping the flap, and trimming the excess mucosa using microinstrumentation are mainstream.[46] The surgical instrumentation includes cold knife and suction,[47] carbon dioxide laser,[48,49] or microdebrider.[1,50] Multiple studies report on the results of each specific technique, but no studies compare the different techniques. Furthermore, an experimental cadaveric model was used to investigate a minimally invasive approach; the authors made a puncture in the cricothyroid membrane or a lateral fenestration in the thyroid cartilage to reach Reinke's space externally with microendoscopes.[51]

Regardless of surgical technique, the dysphonia improves but does not completely normalize.[52] First long-term results showed that the voice was abnormal in 81% of cases postoperatively.[22] The average fundamental frequency in women increases to 150 Hz from 120 Hz, which is still lower than normal and more characteristic of a smoker's voice.[12] (see **Fig. 1**) Therefore, preoperatively patients should be counseled that despite surgical intervention, normalization of the voice is rare.

More recently, office based use of photoangiolytic laser treatment has been investigated. Because the pathophysiology of RE is based on vascular congestion, potassium titanyl phosphate (KTP) laser, which targets oxyhemoglobin, has been employed.

Both can be performed in the office, with minimal risk and avoidance of general anesthesia. Safety, feasibility, and efficiency have been reported in multiple studies.[53–55]

Postoperative management's goal is to reduce risk factors predisposing to recurrence. If surgical techniques are employed, postoperative voice rest is recommended. Postoperative stroboscopic evaluation will likely show persistent mucosal wave abnormalities.[12,46] Postoperative voice therapy is employed to decrease the elevated subglottal pressure seen preoperatively and thus prevent recurrence.[12] Control of reflux and smoking cessation are paramount. Nielsen and colleagues[22] also demonstrated that recurrence was over 58% if smoking cessation was not instituted.

SUMMARY

RE is benign polypoid degeneration of Reinke's space with characteristic histologic, stroboscopic, and aerodynamic findings causing a chief complaint of dysphonia most frequently. Treatment is focused on reducing risk factors, chief of which is smoking cessation, surgically decreasing the polypoid lesion size, and preserving an improved, yet not normal postintervention voice result.

REFERENCES

1. Druck Sant'Anna G, Mauri M. Use of the microdebrider for Reinke's Edema Surgery. Laryngoscope 2000;110(12):2114–6.
2. Hajek M. Anatomische Untersuchungen über das Larynxödem. Langenbecks Arch Chir 1891;42:46–93.
3. Reinke F. Investigation into the human vocal fold. Fortschr Med 1895;12:469–78 [in German].
4. Reinke F. Contributions to the histology of humans part II: on the functional structure of the human vocal folds with special consideration to the elastic tissue. AnatHefte 1897;9:103–7 [in German].
5. Hirano M. Phonosurgery: basic and clinical investigations. Otol Fukouka 1975;21:239–442.
6. Senior A. Friedrich Berthold Reinke (1862–1919): brilliant yet troubled anatomist of the vocal fold. J Laryngol Otol 2015;129(11):1053–7.
7. Hah JH, Sim S, An S-Y, et al. Evaluation of the prevalence of and factors associated with laryngeal diseases among the general population: prevalence of Laryngeal Diseases. Laryngoscope 2015;125(11):2536–42.
8. Lehmann W, Pampurik J, Guyot J-P. Laryngeal pathologies observed in microlaryngoscopy. ORL J Otorhinolaryngol Relat Spec 1989;51(4):206–15.
9. Goswami S, Patra TK. A Clinico-pathological study of Reinke's oedema. Indian J Otolaryngol Head Neck Surg 2003;55(3):160–5.
10. Zeitels SM, Casiano RR, Gardner GM, et al. Management of common voice problems: committee report. Otolaryngol Head Neck Surg 2002;126(4):333–48.
11. Kothe C, Schade G, Fleischer S, et al. Forced inspiration: a laryngoscopy-based maneuver to assess the size of Reinke's edema. Laryngoscope 2003;113(4):741–2.
12. Zeitels SM, Bunting GW, Hillman RE, et al. Reinke's edema: phonatory mechanisms and management strategies. Ann Otol Rhinol Laryngol 1997;106(7):533–43.
13. Tan M, Bryson PC, Pitts C, et al. Clinical grading of Reinke's edema. Laryngoscope 2017;127(10):2310–3.
14. Remenár E, Élö J, Frint T. The morphological basis for development of Reinke's oedema. Acta Otolaryngol 1984;97(1–2):169–76.

15. Sato K, Hirano M, Nakashima T. Electron microscopic and immunohistochemical investigation of Reinke's edema. Ann Otol Rhinol Laryngol 1999;108(11): 1068–72.
16. Hantzakos A, Remacle M, Dikkers FG, et al. Exudative lesions of Reinke's space: a terminology proposal. Eur Arch Otorhinolaryngol 2009;266(6):869–78.
17. Tillmann B, Rudert H, Schünke M, et al. Morphological studies on the pathogenesis of Reinke's edema. Eur Arch Otorhinolaryngol 1995;252(8):469–74.
18. Pastuszek P, Krecicki T, Zalesska-Krecicka M, et al. Histological and electron microscopic investigation of Reinke's edema. Pol J Pathol 2003;54(1):61–4.
19. Sakae FA, Imamura R, Sennes LU, et al. Disarrangement of collagen fibers in Reinke's edema. Laryngoscope 2008;118(8):1500–3.
20. Sakae FA, Imamura R, Sennes LU, et al. Elastic fibers in Reinke's edema. Ann Otol Rhinol Laryngol 2010;119(9):609–14.
21. Gray SD, Hammond E, Hanson DF. Benign pathologic responses of the larynx. Ann Otol Rhinol Laryngol 1995;104(1):13–8.
22. Nielsen VM, Højslet PE, Karlsmose M. Surgical treatment of Reinke's oedema (Long-term results). J Laryngol Otol 1986;100(02):187–90.
23. Marcotullio D, Magliulo G, Pezone T. Reinke's edema and risk factors: clinical and histopathologic aspects. Am J Otolaryngol 2002;23(2):81–4.
24. Myerson MC. Smoker'S Larynx: a clinical pathological entity. Ann Otol Rhinol Laryngol 1950;59(2):541–6.
25. Wallner LJ. Smoker's larynx. Laryngoscope 1954;64(4):259–70.
26. Chung JH, Tae K, Lee YS, et al. The significance of laryngopharyngeal reflux in benign vocal mucosal lesions. Otolaryngol Head Neck Surg 2009;141(3):369–73.
27. Tsikoudas A, Kochillas X, Vernham G. Reinke's oedema, hormones and hormone replacement therapy. J Laryngol Otol 2006;120(10):849–52.
28. Lindeberg H, Felding JU, SøGaard H, et al. Reinke's oedema and thyroid function: a prospective study in 43 patients. Clin Otolaryngol 1987;12(6):417–20.
29. White A, Sim DW, Maran AGD. Reinke's oedema and thyroid function. J Laryngol Otol 1991;105(04):291–2.
30. Woo P, Casper J, Colton R, et al. Dysphonia in the aging: physiology versus disease. Laryngoscope 1992;102(2):139–44.
31. Cohen E, Kolbus A, van Trotsenburg M, et al. Immunohistochemical examinations of sex hormone receptors in benign vocal fold lesions. Folia Phoniatr Logop 2009; 61(5):259–62.
32. Kravos A, Hočevar-Boltežar I, Geršak K. Serum levels of sex hormones in males with Reinke's edema. Eur Arch Otorhinolaryngol 2013;270(1):233–8.
33. Kravos A, Župevc A, Čizmarevič B, et al. The role of allergy in the etiology of Reinke's edema on vocal folds. Wien Klin Wochenschr 2010;122(S2):44–8.
34. Martins RHG, Fabro AT, Domingues MAC, et al. Is Reinke's edema a precancerous lesion? Histological and electron microscopic aspects. J Voice 2009;23(6): 721–5.
35. Moesgaard Nielsen V, Højslet PE, Palvio D. Reinke's oedema: a premalignant condition? J Laryngol Otol 1986;100(10):1159–62.
36. Plch J, Pár I, Navrátilová I, et al. Long term follow-up study of laryngeal precancer. Auris Nasus Larynx 1998;25(4):407–12.
37. Lim S, Sau P, Cooper L, et al. The incidence of premalignant and malignant disease in Reinke's edema. Otolaryngol Head Neck Surg 2014;150(3):434–6.
38. Duflo SM, Thibeault SL, Li W, et al. Differential gene expression profiling of vocal fold polyps and Reinke's edema by complementary DNA microarray. Ann Otol Rhinol Laryngol 2006;115(9):703–14.

39. Branski RC, Saltman B, Sulica L, et al. Cigarette smoke and reactive oxygen species metabolism: Implications for the pathophysiology of Reinke's edema. Laryngoscope 2009;119(10):2014–8.

40. Wang J, Fang R, Peterson A, et al. The protective role of autophagy in human vocal fold fibroblasts under cigarette smoke extract exposure: a new insight into the study of Reinke's edema. ORL J Otorhinolaryngol Relat Spec 2016; 78(1):26–35.

41. Lumpkin SM, Bishop SG, Bennett S. Comparison of surgical techniques in the treatment of laryngeal polypoid degeneration. Ann Otol Rhinol Laryngol 1987; 96(3 Pt 1):254–7.

42. Højslet P-E, Moesgaard-Nielsen V, Karlsmose M. Smoking cessation in chronic Reinke's oedema. J Laryngol Otol 1990;104(08):626–8.

43. Nielsen VM, Højslet P-E. Topical treatment of Reinke's oedema with beclomethasone dipropionate (BDP) inhalation aerosol. J Laryngol Otol 1987;101(09):921–4.

44. Tateya I, Omori K, Kojima H, et al. Steroid injection for Reinke's edema using fiberoptic laryngeal surgery. Acta Otolaryngol 2003;123(3):417–20.

45. Cummings CW, Fredrickson J, Harker L, et al. Benign vocal fold mucosal disorders. In: Otolaryngology—Head and Neck surgery. 3rd edition. St Louis (MO): Mosby; 1998. p. 2096–129.

46. Courey MS, Gardner GM, Stone RE, et al. Endoscopic vocal fold microflap: a three-year experience. Ann Otol Rhinol Laryngol 1995;104(4 Pt 1):267–73.

47. Hirano M, Shin T, Morio M, et al. An improvement in surgical treatment for polypoid vocal cord: sucking technique. Otolagia Fukuoka 1976;(22):583–9.

48. Remacle M, Lawson G, Watelet J-B. Carbon dioxide laser microsurgery of benign vocal fold lesions: indications, techniques, and results in 251 patients. Ann Otol Rhinol Laryngol 1999;108(2):156–64.

49. Murry T, Abitbol J, Hersan R. Quantitative assessment of voice quality following laser surgery for Reinke's edema. J Voice 1999;13(2):257–64.

50. Honda K, Haji T, Maruyama H. Functional results of Reinke's edema surgery using a microdebrider. Ann Otol Rhinol Laryngol 2010;119(1):32–6.

51. Hoffman HT, Bock JM, Karnell LH, et al. Microendoscopy of Reinke's space. Ann Otol Rhinol Laryngol 2008;117(7):510–4.

52. Martins RHG, Tavares ELM, Pessin ABB. Are vocal alterations caused by smoking in Reinke's edema in women entirely reversible after microsurgery and smoking cessation? J Voice 2017;31(3):380.e11-14.

53. Pitman MJ, Lebowitz-Cooper A, Iacob C, et al. Effect of the 532nm pulsed KTP laser in the treatment of Reinke's edema: 532 nm pulsed KTP laser and Reinke's edema. Laryngoscope 2012;122(12):2786–92.

54. Koszewski IJ, Hoffman MR, Young WG, et al. Office-based photoangiolytic laser treatment of Reinke's edema: safety and voice outcomes. Otolaryngol Head Neck Surg 2015;152(6):1075–81.

55. Young VN, Mallur PS, Wong AW, et al. Analysis of potassium titanyl phosphate laser settings and voice outcomes in the treatment of Reinke's edema. Ann Otol Rhinol Laryngol 2015;124(3):216–20.

Vocal Fold Paresis

Chandra M. Ivey, MD*

KEYWORDS

- Vocal fold paresis • Vocal fold paralysis • Vocal fatigue • Glottic incompetence
- Sensory neuropathy • Laryngeal electromyography

KEY POINTS

- Clinical suspicion for paresis should be raised in patients with voice changes, vocal fatigue, difficulty projecting, or pain with voice use.
- Signs of paresis noted on light laryngoscopy include motion abnormalities, bowing atrophy, level difference, and length asymmetries.
- Videostroboscopic signs of paresis include asymmetric mucosal wave, tension asymmetries, phase abnormalities, and evidence of glottic insufficiency.
- Laryngeal electromyography is used as a confirmatory examination after having clinical suspicion for paresis.
- Voice therapy, injection augmentation, and medialization thyroplasty may decrease the glottic incompetence associated with vocal fold paresis and improve symptoms.

DEFINITION OF VOCAL FOLD PARESIS

Vocal fold paresis is the partial impairment of vocal fold motor function that is caused by nerve or neuromuscular abnormality.[1] This partial damage changes glottic closure and efficiency, which contributes to voice impairment. Paresis can be considered separate from vocal fold paralysis, with a distinct set of complaints and findings on examination. The diagnosis of vocal fold paresis has been noted in approximately one-sixth, or 15% of new voice patients presenting to the laryngologist.[2] In many cases the symptoms are rather vague and may be attributed to a laundry list of potential etiologies. One study found that paresis was one of the most commonly missed diagnoses in patients with voice symptoms attributed to laryngopharyngeal reflux.[3] Even the clinical signs leading to suspicion for vocal fold paresis may be varied and subtle, causing doubt in their clinical relevance and often leading to underdiagnosis of this problem.

SIGNIFICANCE OF VOCAL FOLD PARESIS

Traditional evaluation of vocal fold motion sought to differentiate absence of motion, that is, paralysis, from motion. With use of indirect mirror laryngoscopy or direct

Disclosure Statement: The author has nothing to disclose.
Icahn School of Medicine, Mount Sinai Hospital, New York, NY, USA
* 210 East 86th Street, 9th Floor, New York, NY 10028.
E-mail address: chandraivey@yahoo.com

fiberoptic laryngoscopy, motion is still often determined as "present" or "absent." Otolaryngologists have recognized that many patients for whom motion is determined as "present" still have laryngeal complaints. Use of electrophysiology to assess vocal fold paralysis has shown heterogeneity and it has been posited that vocal fold impairment should, in fact, be considered as a continuum.[4]

Completely "perfect" glottic neurologic function includes efferent motor activity that adducts, abducts, and stretches the vocal folds to modulate vocalization, breathing, and subglottic pressure. The motor components of superior laryngeal nerve (SLN) through the external laryngeal nerve are responsible for cricothyroid activity, and the major motor input for the thyroarytenoid (TA) and posterior cricoarytenoid (PCA), along with the other intrinsic muscles of the larynx, is through the recurrent laryngeal nerve (RLN). The afferent neurologic function, which includes chemical, temperature, touch and pain sensation, must also have normal activity to modulate and impact this motor activity (**Fig. 1**). The glossopharyngeal nerve fibers to the vocal folds and surrounding supraglottic structures are also carried through the SLN through the internal laryngeal nerve. The RLN carries the fibers responsible for sensation in the subglottis and trachea. The sympathetic chain also lends fibers to modulate activity in the larynx through these nerves. If there is damage to ANY portion of this neurologic circuit, functional deficit may occur. Patients often complain of altered sensation (ie, tickle, burning, cough, mucus) as well as vocal fatigue or symptoms of muscle tension dysphonia (MTD). These are less well defined when compared with the definitive breathy dysphonia of the traditional vocal fold paralysis with overt vocal fold immobility found on examination.

Those patients with altered but working nerve function are often a conundrum for the otolaryngologist. They are underdiagnosed as being normal, or misdiagnosed as having other conditions like reflux, globus, or primary MTD. The changes in subglottic pressure that may occur with this condition can cause varying degrees of glottic insufficiency that are not identified, yet may still cause vocal and breathing complaints.

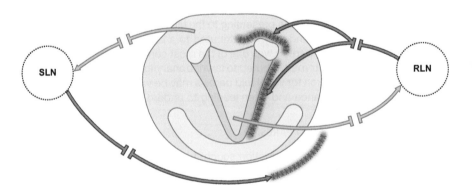

Fig. 1. Afferent and efferent contributions to the SLN and the RLN. Figure displays where alterations in any portions of the afferent or efferent pathways of the SLN and RLN may lead to abnormal motion or sensation causing symptoms and signs of paresis. Sensory inputs have been placed on one side of the larynx and motor has been placed on the other for ease of description but operate ipsilaterally.

Box 1
Possible causes of vocal fold paresis
Anterior cervical discectomy and fusion
Carotid endarterectomy
Cerebrovascular accident
Charcot-Marie-Tooth disease
Chemotherapy
Goiter
Idiopathic
Intubation
Lyme disease
Multiple sclerosis
Myasthenia gravis
Neoplasm
Post-viral
Thyroidectomy
Transient ischemic attack
Trauma
Parkinson syndromes

HISTORY AND PHYSICAL EXAMINATION
Causes for Vocal Fold Paresis

Causes of paresis are similar to those of complete vocal fold paralysis and are included in **Box 1**. Upper respiratory illness, throat pain, or initial cough may be noted to precede vocal symptoms.[5] Paresis is often considered idiopathic, but potentially any pathology present from skull base to mediastinum that compresses, tethers, stretches, or infiltrates contributing fibers to the SLN or RLN may cause abnormalities. Neurologic conditions or insults, such as transient ischemic attack and stroke, may affect vocal fold function and should be assessed if appropriate. History of neck surgery or intubation may be present. Neoplasms involving the head, neck, or chest, as well as benign thyroid disease may affect the laryngeal nerves.

Symptoms of Vocal Fold Paresis

Patients with varying degrees of altered RLN and/or SLN function typically complain of voice changes.[4] They infrequently complain of breathiness, but instead complain of vocal fatigue. This includes breathlessness with speaking, difficulty being heard in noisy environments, decreased vocal range, and instability of the voice with increased use. There may be associated feelings of strain or soreness in the neck with voice use, or even frank pain. Associated cough, globus, and choking sensations also may be present. Potential complaints that may signify paresis and that should be considered when interviewing a patient are listed in **Box 2**. Although patients report similar constellations of symptoms, it is often difficult to quantify their severity. The Voice Handicap Index (VHI) or VHI-10, and the Glottal Function Index are self-assessment scales that help to determine functional severity of voice complaints.[6–8] These have been validated and show improvement with improved voice function, thus are helpful in monitoring treatment response.

Box 2
Possible symptoms of vocal fold paresis

Breathlessness with speech

Breathy voice

Clearing of the throat

Cough

Difficulty in loud environments

Difficulty projecting voice

Globus sensation

Noisy breathing

Pain with speaking

Pitch changes

Pitch restriction

Poor voice in the evenings

Strained voice

Throat pain

Voice fatigue

Voice changes

Signs of Vocal Fold Paresis

The otolaryngologist has useful tools to assist in the diagnosis of vocal fold paresis. Both light laryngoscopy and videostroboscopy are important for determining features of partial weakness. Light laryngoscopy is the most common tool used to diagnose vocal fold paralysis because the overt differential motion is easy to visualize with this technique. This can hold true for paresis, but basic evaluation of motion may not be diagnostic in all cases. Signs of paresis may be categorized as static or dynamic. Static changes are characteristics or asymmetries that can be noted without the vocal fold being in motion. Examples of this are atrophy, bowing, ventricular widening, arytenoid prolapse, and some length asymmetries (**Fig. 2**). Dynamic signs may be seen only while the vocal fold is in motion. These include asymmetric motion,

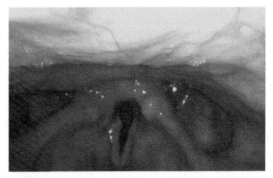

Fig. 2. Light laryngoscopy displaying static signs of paresis: vocal process asymmetry and vocal fold bowing. The vocal process on the right is posterior to that on the left and the right vocal fold shows bowing, both indicative of right vocal fold paresis.

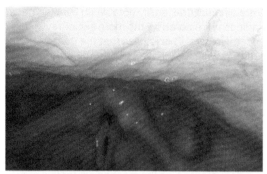

Fig. 3. Light laryngoscopy showing dynamic signs of paresis: vocal fold level difference. The vocal fold on the right is approximating under the left, showing possible vocal fold paresis.

opening or closing, phase shift, supraglottic hyperfunction, height differences, or mucosal wave amplitude asymmetries (**Fig. 3**). Potential signs of vocal fold paresis are organized in this fashion and listed in **Table 1**.

Wu and Sulica[2] surveyed laryngologists to determine which features of the examination were considered diagnostic in each physician's practice. Videostroboscopy was found to be the main tool used for diagnosis instead of light laryngoscopy. It was noted that the diagnosis was not made on any single element, but based on the gestalt history, symptoms, and signs that were noted. Isseroff and colleagues[9] performed systematic investigation to determine which signs indicating paresis were most consistently noted across physician experience levels. The findings with the highest interrater reliability were noted to be shorter vocal fold, thin vocal fold, bowing, reduced motion, and dysdiadochokinesis (asymmetric rapid motion).

Table 1
Possible signs of vocal fold paresis

Static	Dynamic
Arytenoid prolapse or asymmetry	Asymmetric mucosal wave
Asymmetry of the vocal process	Asymmetry of the vocal process
Bowing of the vocal fold[a]	Axis deviation
False fold hypertrophy	Decreased vocal fold motion
Height difference[a]	Differential AB-duction
Laxity of the vocal fold	Differential AD-duction
Length asymmetry[a]	Dysdiadochokinesis
Piriform sinus widening	False fold hypertrophy
Shortening of the vocal fold	Height difference[a]
Thinning (atrophy) of the vocal fold[a]	Phase lag/shift
Ventricular widening	Supraglottic hyperfunction

Signs of paresis may be considered as either static (noted while the vocal fold is at rest) or dynamic (noted while the vocal fold is in motion). At times asymmetries may change or be more apparent during alternating breathing and speaking. Some signs may be noted both during static and dynamic tasks and are listed in both columns.

[a] Indicates the most reliable signs found on laryngoscopy across different levels of experience as determined in Isseroff et al.[9]

Data from Isseroff TF, Parasher AK, Richards A, et al. Interrater reliability in analysis of laryngoscopic features for unilateral vocal fold paresis. J Voice 2016;30(6):736–40.

Interestingly, these are all measures easily notable on light laryngoscopy; some of the key stroboscopic findings were noted by the more senior reviewers but were not used by the less experienced viewers. This implies that the general otolaryngologist will be able to use tools they likely already have in their office to reliably predict vocal fold paresis, and may need to refer to the laryngologist for confirmation and management, not for diagnosis.

Associated Respiratory Symptoms

Patients with vocal fold paresis may present with respiratory or sensory complaints instead of typical vocal fatigue and dysphonia. There may be history of exercise intolerance or dyspnea performing tasks that in the past were without difficulty. Any airway complaints should be documented, as the mechanism for this may be varied. Because vocal fold weakness may cause a variable extrathoracic obstruction, there may be increased resistance while attempting to take in deep or rapid breaths.[10] Some literature is available noting that improving glottic closure with augmentation improves the sensation of dyspnea in some patients.[11]

Alternatively, synkinesis may occur and cause airway obstruction through inappropriate adduction of the abnormal vocal fold during inspiration.[12] This may cause stridor or airway compromise necessitating intervention. This has been shown with laryngeal electromyography (LEMG) by noting increased recruitment of TA muscle activity during breathing maneuvers instead of with speaking maneuvers. Botulinum toxin A has been used to decrease synkinetic activity and improve both stridor and breathing.[13]

Associated Sensory Symptoms

Internal laryngeal nerve or RLN damage may cause sensation changes in the larynx. These are often described in vague terms like urge to cough, coughing spasm, tickle, irritation, feeling of mucus, painful sensation, burning, or dryness.[14] The laryngeal adductor response has been recorded and popularized for sensory testing of the larynx during functional endoscopic evaluation of swallow with sensory testing.[15] Although other sensory testing tools are being investigated, there is no consensus on sensory testing or its role in diagnosis of sensory neuropathy at this time.

Regardless of ability to confirm sensory neuropathy, vigilant avoidance of triggers may improve cough sensation and other sensations of irritation in the throat. Neuromodulating medications have been trialed in off-label fashion for control of sensory symptoms in the larynx.[16] At times, even understanding that some of these unexplained sensations and symptoms may stem from a neuropathy and are not an indication of a deeper or more malignant as-yet-undiagnosed problem offers patients some reassurance.

DIAGNOSTIC TESTING
Computed Tomography

When vocal fold paralysis is noted, computed tomography (CT) is often recommended if no iatrogenic cause is noted. This allows the skull base, neck, and chest to be imaged in search for a potential cause for the nerve damage. It is important to recognize that use of CT in cases of paresis has not been shown to be helpful.[17] Badia and colleagues[17] retrospectively investigated 81 cases of unilateral vocal fold paresis and ultimately found a 0% positive rate for identifying causative pathology using this test. This is in contrast to a fair rate of return for use of CT for idiopathic paralysis, listed at between 35% and 55%.[18,19]

Laryngeal Electromyography

Currently, LEMG is the test of choice for confirmation of vocal fold paresis. The use of this tool for diagnosis of vocal fold paralysis has been more extensively studied, but a few studies distinctly reporting on its utility for hypomobility have been published.[20–23] Routine testing of bilateral TA and cricothyroid muscles, and selective testing of PCA muscles is common when performing LEMG. Heman-Ackah and Barr[23] compiled data from patients with clinical evidence of paresis where electromyography (EMG) had been performed.[23] Activity parameters that were tested are listed in **Box 3**. Neuropathy was confirmed if decreased recruitment, increased motor unit action potential (MUAP) amplitude, and/or polyphasic MUAPs were present. Eighty-six percent of patients suspected of having paresis on clinical examination had positive confirmation of this by LEMG. More than half of the patients were found to have bilateral paresis based on the strict criteria used in this study. It was noted that no specific pattern of muscle activity found on examination could accurately predict the pattern of abnormality noted on LEMG. Although the clinician could adequately predict that there was asymmetry and likely paresis, the site and side was not always correlated by the EMG data. This observation has been supported by other similar studies.[24] Use of LEMG for confirmation of vocal fold paresis has been criticized because of these factors. It is also criticized because decreased MUAP recruitment, one of the most common abnormal findings to diagnose paresis, also may be attributed to decreased patient effort, making it less specific. Many clinicians also feel that LEMG is still qualitative, so therefore cannot be used for confirmation. Effort is being made to systematize LEMG so that its use may be more wholeheartedly accepted to diagnose this condition.

NATURAL HISTORY OF PARESIS

There has been no study of the prevalence of asymptomatic vocal fold paresis in the general population. An idea of how prevalent this is in an asymptomatic cohort would offer better understanding of asymmetries in vocal fold mobility in general, as well as allow for study of the differences between patients who show functional deficits and those who do not. There are also no studies published specifically on the natural history or recovery after vocal fold partial paralysis. It is thought that most patients likely resolve without treatment because their symptoms are mild or vague. Extrapolation from recent studies on idiopathic vocal fold paralysis may offer some potential benchmarks.[25] This showed that 69% of symptomatic patients recovered function within 6 months of onset. Patients with vocal fold paresis often go undiagnosed for many months and are more likely to be treated as primary muscle tension or reflux-related dysphonia without significant improvement. It has previously been noted that

---

Box 3
Laryngeal electromyography (LEMG) parameters for vocal fold paresis*

Insertional activity

Motor unit action potential (MUAP) amplitude

MUAP duration

MUAP morphology

Recruitment pattern

Synkinetic activity

* As noted in Heman-Ackah and Barr.[23]

approximately 1 in 6, or 15% of new laryngology visits are thought to have paresis.[2] It may be that the patients who are finally coming to the laryngologist are those who have not shown functional improvement with time, and thus they will need more aggressive therapy or intervention. Further study to elucidate how common this problem is, how severe denervation must be to elicit functional deficit, and the natural time course for recovery must be initiated.

VOICE THERAPY FOR VOCAL FOLD PARESIS

Most of the voice symptoms present with vocal fold paresis are thought to occur due to glottic incompetence. Because the tone or motion of the affected vocal fold is inadequate, this generates altered subglottic pressure, flow, and dyssynchronous mucosal wave propagation that leads to poor projection of the voice or lack of stability over time. Compensatory maneuvers of the unaffected vocal fold or other intrinsic muscles of the larynx, as well abnormal recruitment of the extrinsic vocal fold muscles occurs to improve the voice stability. This may lead to secondary MTD, the major symptoms of which are vocal strain, worsening voice or fatigue over time, and potential pain with voice use. Voice therapy is recommended for patients with these symptoms as first-line therapy.[26] Goals of this intervention are to dispel dysfunctional compensation in favor of more functional techniques for improving subglottic pressure and flow characteristics. Patients often respond favorably to these exercises and rebalancing of the vocal system, despite the fact that therapy does not intrinsically change the denervation that has occurred.

Speech language pathologists are trained in multifactorial approaches to MTD and are able to spend time assessing nonmedical factors that may also affect dysphonia.[27] This may include psychological factors or stressors in the patient's environment that may be impeding optimal voice use. Vocal hygiene routines, if not already implemented by the physician, are used to maximize hydration and lubrication, and adjuncts like microphones, whistles, or other tools are recommended when appropriate. Manual decompression techniques like circumlaryngeal massage to relieve muscle tightness are also used. These changes may assist in developing improved voice use techniques and more functional voicing.

Voice therapy has been shown to help some of the dyspnea and urge to cough symptoms that may accompany vocal fold paresis. Respiratory retraining may decrease stridor noted from inappropriate vocal fold motion, and may improve some dyspnea by retraining breathing and speaking coordination.

ADJUVANTS FOR SENSORY NEUROPATHY AND BREATHING ABNORMALITIES

As previously mentioned, medical therapy may be indicated for some of the associated sensory or breathing abnormalities accompanying vocal fold paresis. Trials of gabapentin and pregabalin have been published showing positive symptom control of cough due to sensory neuropathy.[28] These neuromodulators seem to have greater effect in patients with chronic cough that also show laryngeal signs of paresis.[29] The effective dose varies and utility is often limited by side effects of fatigue, dizziness, and nausea. A recent meta-analysis was able to show positive effects of gabapentin, baclofen, and amitriptyline on neurogenic cough, but no single mechanism by which all 3 classes of drugs influence neuropathic symptoms was found.[30] Amitriptyline has been shown to be more effective than codeine cough suppressants for neuropathic cough in a prospective randomized controlled study.[31] This medication is often first-line medical therapy for symptoms of neurogenic cough or urge to cough sensation. One older study has been published on use of baclofen to increase cough threshold with promising effects.[32] It is important to remember these studies are publishing off-label uses of medications in small numbers of subjects, so should not be taken as standard of care.

Botulinum toxin A has been used to decrease stridor and dyspnea in conditions such as paradoxic vocal fold motion, unilateral and bilateral vocal fold paralysis, and focal dystonia.[33] This has also been used with positive results in chronic cough.[34] Treatment efficacy is likely due to weakening of the adductor ability of the TA muscle that then leads to weaker cough and less airway obstruction during inspiration. This treatment is used to prevent surgical intervention, such as cordotomy or tracheotomy, in borderline cases of airway obstruction. Botulinum toxin A use in the larynx is also off-label but is considered standard of care in cases of laryngeal dystonia. This treatment is not considered gold standard for dyspnea or symptomatic synkinesis.

SURGICAL INTERVENTION FOR VOCAL FOLD PARESIS

Surgical intervention for glottic incompetence may be necessary if patients continue to be symptomatic after a trial of voice therapy. These procedures are germane to improving glottic closure, and are used regardless of the cause for the decreased strength of closure, whether from vocal fold paresis, bowing atrophy, presbylaryngeus, or vocal fold paralysis.

Injection Augmentation

Injection augmentation was popularized with the introduction of Teflon in the 1960s and was used to close large vocal fold gaps from vocal fold paralysis.[35] This procedure was straightforward and could even be performed in the office setting once fiberoptic technology became widely available.[36] Teflon injection fell out of favor over time due to inflammatory foreign body reaction that detrimentally affected the vibratory features of the larynx and caused large granuloma formation that could obstruct the airway. Other injectable materials are now available and are considered safe, so there has been a significant resurgence in the popularity of this procedure. **Box 4** includes many of the available injectable materials commonly used at this time.

Box 4
Materials currently available for injection augmentation

Autologous fascia

Autologous fat

Bioplastique

Bovine-derived collagen

Calcium hydroxylapatite

Carboxymethylcellulose

Gel carrier

Gelfoam

Human-derived fibroblasts

Hyaluronic acid derivatives

Micronized AlloDerm

(Teflon)

Laryngeal Framework Surgery

Medialization thyroplasty has been commonly used for the improvement of glottic incompetence, and thus may be beneficial for symptomatic vocal fold paresis. Silastic and hydroxylappetite rigid implants are common for intervention in paralysis and have been extrapolated for use even when the vocal folds are mobile. Expanded polytetra-fluoroethylene (Gore-Tex) is a softer implant that has been popularized in the early 2000s.[37] It is important to note that there typically is no role for arytenoid relocation procedures during framework surgery for paresis, as the vocal fold and joint are mobile.

Laryngeal Reinnervation

Because the vocal folds are mobile in cases of symptomatic vocal fold paresis, there has been no noted role for laryngeal reinnervation. This procedure severs the nonfunctional RLN in order to improve tone by reconnecting the distal portion to a more functional nerve. Vocal fold paresis, by definition, implies at least a partially mobile vocal fold, so any further trauma to the nerve should be avoided.

SUMMARY

Vocal fold paresis is abnormal neuromotor function that is diagnosed when patients complain of vocal fatigue, difficulty projecting, pain with speaking, and hoarseness, but have mobile vocal folds. Constellations of signs and symptoms have been reviewed with the goal of familiarizing physicians on the nuances of diagnosis for paresis. Associated respiratory and sensory deficits commonly noted have been reviewed and should be documented and treated when appropriate. Current therapies including voice therapy, surgical intervention for persistent glottic incompetence, and adjuvant therapies for concurrent sensory neuropathy and synkinesis are described. Most importantly, a high level of suspicion for potential paresis is recommended for patients who have complaints suggestive of glottic incompetence regardless of overt mobility of the vocal folds.

REFERENCES

1. Blitzer A, Crumley RL, Dailey SH, et al. Recommendations of the neurolaryngology study group on laryngeal electromyography. Otolaryngol Head Neck Surg 2009;140:782–93.
2. Wu AP, Sulica L. Diagnosis of vocal fold paresis: current opinion and practice. Laryngoscope 2015;125:904–8.
3. Rafii B, Taliercio S, Achlatis S, et al. Incidence of underlying laryngeal pathology in patients initially diagnosed with laryngopharyngeal reflux. Laryngoscope 2014; 124:1420–4.
4. Sulica L, Blitzer A. Vocal fold paresis: evidence and controversies. Curr Opin Otolaryngol Head Neck Surg 2007;15:159–62.
5. Koufman JA, Postma GN, Cummins MM, et al. Vocal fold paresis. Otolaryngol Head Neck Surg 2000;122:537–41.
6. Jacobson BH, Johnson A, Grimalkin C, et al. The voice handicap index (VHI): development and validation. Am J Speech Lang Pathol 1997;6:66–70.
7. Rosen CA, Lee AS, Osborne J, et al. Development and validation of the voice handicap index-10. Laryngoscope 2004;114:1549–56.
8. Bach KK, Belafsky PC, Wasylik K, et al. Validity and reliability of the glottal function index. Arch Otolaryngol Head Neck Surg 2005;131:961–4.

9. Isseroff TF, Parasher AK, Richards A, et al. Interrater reliability in analysis of lar-yngoscopic features for unilateral vocal fold paresis. J Voice 2016;30(6):736–40.
10. Cantarella G, Fasano V, Bucchioni E, et al. Variability of specific airway resistance in patients with laryngeal hemiplegia. Ann Otol Rhinol Laryngol 2005;114:434–8.
11. Dion GR, Fritz MA, Teng SE, et al. Impact of vocal fold augmentation and laryng-oplasty on dyspnea in patients with glottal incompetence. Laryngoscope 2017; 128:427–9.
12. Woo P, Mangaro M. Aberrant recurrent laryngeal nerve reinnervation as a cause of stridor and laryngospasm. Ann Otol Rhinol Laryngol 2004;113(10):805–8.
13. Lekue A, Garcia-Lopez I, Santiago S, et al. Diagnosis and management with bot-ulinum toxin in 11 cases of laryngeal synkinesis. Eur Arch Otorhinolaryngol 2015; 272:2397–402.
14. Lee B, Woo P. Chronic cough as a sign of laryngeal sensory neuropathy: diag-nosis and treatment. Ann Otol Rhinol Laryngol 2005;114:253–7.
15. Aviv J. Clinical assessment of pharyngolaryngeal sensitivity. Am J Med 2000; 108(4A):68S–72S.
16. Altman KW, Noordzij P, Rosen C, et al. Neurogenic cough. Laryngoscope 2015; 125:1675–81.
17. Badia PI, Hillel AT, Shah MD, et al. Computed tomography has low yield in the evaluation of idiopathic unilateral true vocal paresis. Laryngoscope 2013;123: 204–7.
18. Terris DJ, Arnstein D, Nguyen HH. Contemporary evaluation of unilateral vocal cord paralysis. Otolaryngol Head Neck Surg 1992;107:84–90.
19. Ramadan JJ, Wax M, Avery S. Outcome and changing course of unilateral vocal cord paralysis. Otolaryngol Head Neck Surg 1998;118:199–202.
20. Blair RL, Berry H, Briant TDR. Laryngeal electromyography: techniques and application. Otolaryngol Clin North Am 1978;11:325–46.
21. Miller RH, Rosenfield DB. The role of electromyography in clinical laryngology. Otolaryngol Head Neck Surg 1984;92:287–91.
22. Haglund S, Knutsson E, Martensson A. An electromyographic analysis of idio-pathic vocal cord paresis. Acta Otolaryngol 1972;74:265–70.
23. Heman-Ackah Y, Barr A. Mild vocal fold paresis: understanding clinical presenta-tion and electromyographic findings. J Voice 2006;20(2):269–81.
24. Simpson CB, Cheung EJ, Jackson CJ. Vocal fold paresis: clinical and electro-physiologic features in a tertiary laryngology practice. J Voice 2009;23:396–8.
25. Husain S, Sadoughi B, Mor N, et al. Time course of recovery of idiopathic vocal fold paralysis. Laryngoscope 2018;128:148–52.
26. MacKenzie K, Millar A, Wilson JA, et al. Is voice therapy an effective treatment for dysphonia? A randomized controlled trial. Br Med J 2001;323:658–61.
27. Van Houtte E, Van Lierde K, Claeys S. Pathophysiology and treatment of muscle tension dysphonia: a review of the current knowledge. J Voice 2011;25(2):202–7.
28. Halum SL, Sycamore DL, McRae BR. A new treatment option for laryngeal sen-sory neuropathy. Laryngoscope 2009;119:1844–7.
29. Giliberto JP, Dibildox D, Merati A. Unilateral laryngoscopic findings associated with response to gabapentin in patients with chronic cough. JAMA Otolaryngol Head Neck Surg 2017;143(11):1081–5.
30. Wei W, Liu R, Tong YZ, et al. The efficacy of specific neuromodulators on human refractory chronic cough: a systematic review and meta-analysis. J Thorac Dis 2016;8(10):2942–51.

31. Jeyakumar A, Brickman TM, Haben M. Effectiveness of amitriptyline versus cough suppressants in the treatment of chronic cough resulting from postviral vagal neuropathy. Laryngoscope 2006;116:2108–12.
32. Dicpinigaitis PV, Rauf K. Treatment of chronic cough with baclofen. Respiration 1998;65:86–8.
33. Woisard V, Liu X, Arne Bes MC, et al. Botulinum toxin injection in laryngeal dyspnea. Eur Arch Otorhinolaryngol 2017;274:909–17.
34. Sasieta HC, Iyer VN, Orbelo DM, et al. Bilateral thyroarytenoid botulinum toxin type A injection for the treatment of refractory chronic cough. JAMA Otolaryngol Head Neck Surg 2016;142(9):881–8.
35. Arnold GE. Vocal rehabilitation of paralytic dysphonia, IX. Technique of intracordal injection. Arch Otolaryngol 1962;76:358–68.
36. Chu PY, Chang SY. Transoral Teflon injection under flexible laryngovideostroboscopy for unilateral vocal fold paralysis. Ann Otol Rhinol Laryngol 1997;106:783–6.
37. McCulloch TM, Hoffman HT. Medialization laryngoplasty with expanded polytetrafluoroethylene: surgical technique and preliminary results. Ann Otol Rhinol Laryngol 1998;107:427–32.

Voice Therapy as Primary Treatment of Vocal Fold Pathology

Wendy DeLeo LeBorgne, BFA, MA, PhD, CCC-SLP[a,b,c,]*,
Erin Nicole Donahue, BM, MA, CCC-SLP[a,b]

KEYWORDS

- Voice therapy • Vocal fold pathology • Dysphonia • Efficacy • Treatment

KEY POINTS

- Voice therapy may provide an effective nonsurgical treatment option for benign vocal fold pathology.
- Efficacy data regarding multiple voice therapy modalities are reviewed in this article.
- Preoperative and postoperative voice therapy has been shown efficacious for optimal phonosurgical outcomes.
- Team decision making (otolaryngologist, speech pathologist, and patient) is essential for compliance, therapeutic progress, and recovery.

INTRODUCTION

Voice therapy contributes to increased effectiveness and efficiency in the otolaryngologist's diagnosis and treatment of voice disorders. Research data and expert clinical experience support the use of voice therapy in the management of patients with acute and chronic voice disorders and may obviate surgery. When surgery is necessary, adjuvant voice therapy can improve surgical outcomes, prevent additional injury, and limit additional treatment costs.[1]

Akin to physical therapy for the treatment of nonsurgical or presurgical physical injuries, voice therapy is a nonmedical, nonsurgical approach to treatment of voice disorders. A voice disorder as defined by multiple sources and published on the American Speech-Language-Hearing Association (ASHA): "occurs when voice

Disclosure Statement: The Authors have nothing to disclose.
[a] The Blaine Block Institute for Voice Analysis and Rehabilitation, 1222 South Patterson Boulevard, Dayton, OH 45402, USA; [b] The Professional Voice Center of Greater Cincinnati, 2123 Auburn Avenue, Suite 315, Cincinnati, OH 45219, USA; [c] University of Cincinnati, CCM/TAPAA, Musical Theater, PO Box 210003, Cincinnati, OH 45221-0003, USA
* Corresponding author. The Blaine Block Institute for Voice Analysis and Rehabilitation, 1222 South Patterson Boulevard, Dayton, OH 45402, USA
E-mail address: wleborgne@soents.com

Otolaryngol Clin N Am 52 (2019) 649–656
https://doi.org/10.1016/j.otc.2019.03.009
oto.theclinics.com
0030-6665/19/© 2019 Elsevier Inc. All rights reserved.

quality, pitch, and loudness differ or are inappropriate for an individual's age, gender, cultural background, or geographic location. A voice disorder is present when an individual expresses concern about having an abnormal voice that does not meet daily needs—even if others do not perceive it as different or deviant."[2] The treatment of voice disorders through voice therapy includes remediation of inappropriate neuromotor patterns, restoration of voice function, and prevention of vocal disability. Implementation of voice therapy techniques should be provided only by a certified speech-language pathologist who has undergone specialized training in the evaluation and treatment of voice disorders.

Voice therapy may be used as the primary treatment of a voice disorder or within a broader context using a multidisciplinary approach (medical, surgical, and therapeutic interventions) to management pending the nature and type of voice disorder. The American Academy of Otolaryngology–Head and Neck Surgery (AAO) recommends voice therapy as the primary treatment of muscle tension dysphonia and recognizes voice therapy as an important component in the treatment of various voice disorders and pathologies.[3] Voice therapy as the primary treatment of benign laryngeal pathology has been shown to improve voice handicap and overall outcomes.[4–6] Regarding voice therapy for vocal fold pathology, the AAO states:

> Benign vocal fold lesions are a common cause of dysphonia. Many studies document excellent outcome after voice therapy in patients with a variety of benign lesions. In cases in which surgery is necessary, pre- and post-operative voice therapy may shorten the postoperative recovery time, allowing faster return to work and limiting scar and permanent dysphonia.[3]

This article provides an overview of the history of voice therapy within the context of treatment of laryngeal disorders, types of voice therapy, and efficacy and outcome data to support the use of voice therapy as well as clinical considerations and caveats.

HISTORY OF VOICE THERAPY

Early voice therapy, designed to correct deviant voice, was first reported in the literature in the 1930s. It was derived primarily from vocal habilitation (vs rehabilitation) practices, emerging from training exercises used for singers and speakers. These exercises typically included tasks to optimize respiration, dynamic control, vocal flexibility, and vocal agility and to promote relaxation during sound production.[5–9] Consistent with historical vocal pedagogy techniques, many of the early objectives in vocal rehabilitation continued to be important to address within the context of voice therapy. With time and scientific advancement, however, increased understanding of laryngeal anatomy and physiology and development of aerodynamic and acoustic analysis of voice, laryngeal imaging techniques, wound healing, phonosurgical advancements, and applied motor learning/exercise physiology, voice therapy has resulted in targeted and efficacious treatment of laryngeal disorders.[5,6] Multiple approaches to voice therapy exist, as do specific exercises and techniques that have been developed over time, resulting in specific lines of research to document efficacy for use of given therapy techniques for specified voice disorders. For further insights into the historical roots of voice therapy, readers are provided with additional references at the end of this article.

TYPES OF VOICE THERAPY

Voice therapy may be grouped into 2 primary categories: indirect or direct.[7,10] Indirect voice therapy (IVT) typically consists of counseling and patient education regarding behaviors that can be adjusted and modified to facilitate positive change in the voice (eg, vocal hygiene counseling, hydration recommendation, and use of amplification). Direct voice therapy (DVT) refers to clinician driven and active patient participation through attending voice therapy sessions, during which the patient engages in therapeutic exercises (eg, direct techniques, manual therapies, resonant voice therapy [RVT], vocal function exercises [VFEs], flow phonation, phonation resistance training exercises, and Lee Silverman Voice Treatment). DVT aims to modify and change neuromotor programming for optimal voice production and can be considered akin to the work done in physical therapy. Combined IVT and DVT typically yields optimal outcomes because it integrates behavioral and neurophysiologic change in the voice-disordered patient.[11–21] IVT and DVT may be differentiated further via multiple treatment modalities and specific execution of those treatments. Although there is no consensus on categorization of voice therapy taxonomy, Stemple and colleagues[7] have described 5 subdivisions within IVT and DVT and a brief, descriptive overview of each is provided:

- Hygienic voice therapy (HVT)
- Symptomatic voice therapy (SVT)
- Psychogenic voice therapy (PsVT)
- Physiologic voice therapy (PhVT)
- Eclectic voice therapy (EVT)

HVT endeavors to modify and optimize a patient's vocal hygiene practices.[7,8] HVT generally consists of increasing a patient's knowledge of behaviors that may contribute to development or perpetuation of vocal symptoms. Changes to facilitate modification or elimination of the actions that have a negative impact on voice are the focus of HVT. HVT includes education regarding anatomy and physiology associated with respiration, phonation, and resonance as well as instruction in vocal hygiene practices. Vocal hygiene education is beneficial for patients with voice-related complaints, whether or not the patient plans to attend DVT sessions. Increased knowledge of behaviors and habits that negatively affect vocal production can serve only to improve the vocal health practices of the patient.[18] Furthermore, studies have revealed positive reactions in subjects who have undergone vocal hygiene training, even when changes in patient behaviors were not evident.[11]

SVT directly targets voice-related symptoms (ie, changing frequency of phonation, direct modification of vocal quality, elimination of hard glottal attacks, and reduction of loudness) to improve the overall voice. For example, if a patient presents to the clinic with rough hoarseness secondary to decreased breath support, an SVT approach to treatment may incorporate direct modification of airflow, resulting in improved parameters of vocal fold vibration and thus improved vocal quality and potential resolution of the symptom.

PsVT focuses on the psychosocial and emotional underpinnings of voice disorders. PsVT is warranted in cases of voice disorders with etiologies related to psychological stress or emotion including, but not limited to, muscle tension dysphonia and functional (conversion) voice disorders. Aspects of PsVT include extensive interviewing and counseling. If a patient's vocal symptoms do not improve given this approach and/or the emotional reason for the voice disorder is beyond the scope of practice of a speech-language pathologist, referral to a mental health professional (psychiatrist and/or psychologist) may be warranted to treat the underlying emotional or psychosocial problem.

PhVT consists of physiologic-based exercises designed to train and rebalance the subsystems of voice to improve vocal quality. Lines of research supporting the efficacy of these techniques are discussed later. PhVT exercises are designed using principles of exercise physiology and motor learning to maximize strength and efficiency in the respiratory (inspiratory muscle strength training, and expiratory muscle strength training), phonotory (VFEs, phonation resistance training exercises, and Lee Silverman Voice Treatment), and resonance (RVT and semioccluded vocal tract exercises).[22–24] Using Specific Adaptation to Imposed Demands principles found in the exercise physiology literature, many of these techniques have excellent data to support utilization for maximized patient care and recovery. Manual laryngeal therapy (eg, circumlaryngeal massage, laryngeal reposturing, and myofascial release) also falls under the category of PhVT because it is a hands-on, directed approach to modify and change suboptimal respiration, voice, and/or whole-body muscular tightness or fascial restrictions impeding typical voice production. PhVT becomes an important part of voice therapy because it gives patients something positive and active "to do" about their voice problem as opposed to only providing a "do not do" list of recommendations (eg, do not yell, do not eat foods that cause reflux, and do not drink caffeine).

EVT incorporates many, if not all, of the aforementioned categories of voice therapy. EVT provides a comprehensive approach to successful voice therapy because it includes a varied, yet targeted, approach to treatment of a given voice disorder. For a given vocally enthusiastic, phonotraumatic patient presenting to the voice clinic with vocal fold nodules, the following example is provided for consideration of integration of EVT. Initially, an HVT approach would aim to improve hydration practices, reduction of vocal dose, and load as well as elimination of phonotraumatic behaviors. PhVT integrates targeted exercises to rebalance respiration, phonation, and resonance through a series of structured exercises the patient learns and subsequently performs at home on a daily basis, ultimately changing suboptimal patterns for optimal neuromotor voice production. Modification of abhorrent vocal symptoms contributing to the vocal pathology, such as hard glottal attacks or glottal fry, may be addressed through SVT. Finally, emotional aspects (eg, "people know me by my husky voice and I like that" or "I'm under so much stress at home/work/school that I can't do my job because of my voice") that are having a negative impact on voice would be addressed through PsVT.

Duration of therapy session, frequency of therapy intervals, and overall length of the therapy process are varied across centers, settings, and regions of the country. Patient compliance, therapist competence, nature of vocal fold pathology, concurrent medical/surgical management, and breadth/depth of exercises incorporated into the course of DVT are considerations for duration, frequency, and length of successful voice therapy.[25,26] A 2015 study revealed the average length of treatment as approximately 10.87 voice therapy sessions over the course of 9.25 weeks, most often occurring once to twice per week, according to an analysis of scholarly articles published between 1975 and 2013. Furthermore, this study noted an average of 8.17 total hours of DVT for patients with various vocal pathologies.[25]

EFFICACY OF VOICE THERAPY

Initial efficacy data regarding voice therapy outcomes date back to the 1940s and were primarily case studies and anecdotal reports of improvement. As voice therapy techniques were refined and instrumental assessment of voice improved in the 1980s and 1990s, there was an increase in the number of studies documenting the benefit of voice therapy in the treatment of voice disorders. Further development of voice therapy techniques through current day has resulted in specific lines of research and treatment modalities for various voice disorders and pathologies.[4,5]

ASHA has created a rigorous systematic review of treatment and efficacy data through an evidence-based mapping and rating system (https://www.asha.org/evidence-maps/). Of relevance regarding recent findings, the following references indicate improvement of voice and laryngeal pathology without surgical intervention:

1. Yiu and colleagues[22] provided data from 9 studies yielding improvement in glottal efficiency through RVT.
2. Angadi and colleagues[23] reviewed 21 research articles regarding the use of VFEs, with the results of the studies demonstrating improvement in vocal function through the use of VFEs.
3. Ribeiro and colleagues[24] present a review of studies on the use of laryngeal manual therapy techniques for voice disorders.

Strong efficacy data continue to emerge for the use of voice therapy as a viable primary option for treatment of select laryngeal pathologies in both pediatric and adult patient populations. "Previous studies found that 21.1% to 56.3% improvement and 38% disappearance of vocal fold polyps could be achieved after conservative treatment with voice therapy. In cases of vocal fold nodules, some researchers achieved elimination or reduction of the lesions in 23% to 81.8% of patients."[18(p2)] Even in cases of the vocal fold lesion persisting on completion of voice therapy, significant positive changes in patient self-assessment measures have been noted.[22]

Additionally, in cases of surgery that is warranted or likely required, a short course (2–4 weeks) of preoperative voice therapy may maximize surgical outcome for the laryngologist by (1) elimination of contributing phonotraumatic behaviors and maximizing vocal hygiene habits, (2) initiation of the process of neuromotor replanning, and (3) optimization of laryngeal tissue status (preoperatively) to promote less invasive surgical techniques and minimize wound creation resulting in decreased postoperative recovery time. Postoperatively, voice therapy may be efficacious to provide patients who have had positive surgical results with an approach to rebuild and rebalance all the subsystems of voice (respiration, phonation, and resonance), similar to postoperative physical therapy. Although there is limited prospective research in the specific area regarding efficacy outcomes after phonosurgery with combined postsurgical voice rehabilitation at this time, there is ample literature in the exercise physiology, physical therapy, and orthopedic literature, which indicates the significant benefit of postoperative therapy approaches, which may parallel the current paradigm of treatment in voice therapy with respect to full return to functional communication status.

THE TEAM APPROACH

A collaborative team approach to injury prevention, treatment, and rehabilitation has proved effective across disciplines. Within the realm of laryngeal pathologies and voice disorders, a comprehensive approach to care is recommended for optimal patient compliance and outcomes. Regardless of setting (university clinic, private practice, or medical model), the primary team members should include an otolaryngologist (with preference for laryngology training) and a certified speech-language pathologist (with preference for a clinician trained in voice and upper airway disorders). As of this writing, Special Interest Group 3, Voice and Voice Disorders, within ASHA currently is in the second phase of consideration for application for board specialty certification in Voice and Upper Airway Disorders. Ancillary team members and specialty practitioners who may be beneficial for full remediation of a patient with laryngeal pathology include gastroenterologist, pulmonologist, psychologist, psychiatrist, physical therapist, and singing voice specialist (a singing teacher with extended training and understanding of voice disorders in a singing population). This list is by no means exhaustive but a consideration of starting point for maximal efficacy of voice therapy.

CONSIDERATIONS AND CAVEATS FOR VOICE THERAPY

Important details to consider when determining whether or not voice therapy is appropriate as the primary treatment of laryngeal pathology include full team evaluation and collaborative planning. During the comprehensive voice assessment (self-rating scales, laryngeal imaging, and aerodynamic and acoustic testing), the following measures should be considered: size and nature of the laryngeal pathology; severity of compromise in amplitude of vibration and mucosal wave as assessed via videostroboscopy at low, comfortable, and high frequencies; and functional communication compromise to the patient in occupational and social settings. Assessment of supraglottic involvement (extrinsic laryngeal muscle involvement) during phonation under various conditions also aid a voice care team in targeting voice therapy to provide optimal outcomes. Respiratory patterns and compensations for laryngeal pathology are vital for treatment planning.

Some specific types of pathology and/or lesions, such as submucosal cysts, do not often respond well to voice therapy as primary treatment, although no efficacy studies regarding this specific pathology were noted in the literature. Voice therapy in these cases, however, may be beneficial to be utilized preoperatively to target behaviors that may result in compromised postoperative healing. Additionally, voice therapy may be beneficial to aid in reduction of acute edema and erythema that can make it difficult to thoroughly assess a vocal fold lesion. Factors, including patient preference and individual time constraints for a particular patient, may influence whether a trial course of DVT should be applied prior to determining whether or not surgical management is warranted or required. In these cases, a short course (2–6 weeks) of DVT may be recommended followed by revisualization and assessment to determine the best course of treatment. Voice therapy is contraindicated for lesions that appear suspicious in nature. Noncancerous lesions, such as leukoplakia, papillomatosis, hyperkeratosis, and parakeratosis, often benefit from postbiopsy voice therapy to promote improved glottic closure and flexibility, thus optimizing functional vocal output.

Just as there is no one size fits all for phonomicrosurgery, optimal surgical outcomes are a combination of specific surgical technique used partnered with a given surgeon's skill set. Similarly, for optimal outcomes in voice therapy, it becomes the joint understanding of the voice therapist to provide the most appropriate therapy technique for a given patient paired with the technical ability for the therapist to deliver the given therapy optimally and appropriately.

REFERENCES

1. Position statement: voice therapy in the treatment of dysphonia. American Academy of Otolaryngology – Head and Neck Surgery; 2016. Available at: https://www.entnet.org//content/voice-therapy-treatment-dysphonia. Accessed September 12, 2018.
2. Voice disorders. American Speech-Language Hearing Association Practice Portal. Available at: https://www.asha.org/Practice-Portal/Clinical-Topics/Voice-Disorders/. Accessed September 12, 2018.
3. Consensus statement on the use of voice therapy in the treatment of dysphonia. American Academy of Otolaryngology – Head and Neck Surgery;

2005. Available at: https://www.entnet.org//content/consensus-statement-use-voice-therapy-treatment-dysphonia. Accessed September 12, 2018.

4. Desjardins M, Halstead L, Cooke M, et al. A systematic review of voice therapy: what "effectiveness" really implies. J Voice 2017;31(3):392.e13-32.

5. Thomas L. The history of outcomes research in voice therapy. Live Presentation (Proceedings) at ASHA Convention. Miami, November 16–18, 2006.

6. Thomas L, Stemple J. Voice therapy: does science support the art? Communicative Disorders Review 2007;1(1):49–77.

7. Stemple J, Roy N, Klaben B. Clinical voice pathology: theory and management. 6th edition. San Diego (CA): Plural Publishing; 2018.

8. Stemple J, Hapner E. Voice therapy: clinical case studies. 5th edition. San Diego (CA): Plural Publishing; 2018.

9. Wendler J. Voice therapy: from the past to the present from a phoniatrician's perspective (Voice of Experience Keynote, PEVOC 2013, Prague). Logoped Phoniatr Vocol 2015;40(2):58–65.

10. Van Stan J, Roy N, Awan S, et al. A taxonomy of voice therapy. Am J Speech Lang Pathol 2015;24:101–25.

11. Broaddus-Lawrence P, Treole K, McCabe R, et al. The effects of preventative vocal hygiene education on the vocal hygiene habits and perceptual vocal characteristics of training singer. J Voice 2000;14(1):58–71.

12. Watts CR. Behavioral voice therapy in school-age children with vocal fold nodules. EBP Briefs 2012;6:1–7.

13. Anderson T, Sataloff R. The power of voice therapy. Ear Nose Throat J 2002;81: 433–4.

14. Holmberg E, Hillman R, Hammarberg B, et al. Efficacy of a behaviorally based voice therapy protocol for vocal nodules. J Voice 2001;15:395–412.

15. Lancer M, Syder D, Jones A, et al. The outcome of different management patterns for vocal cord nodules. J Laryngol Otol 1988;102:423–32.

16. McCrory E. Voice therapy outcomes in vocal fold nodules: a retrospective audit. Int J Lang Commun Disord 2001;36:19–24.

17. Speyer R, Wieneke G, Dejonckere P. Documentation of progress in voice therapy: perceptual, acoustic, and laryngostroboscopic findings pretherapy and posttherapy. J Voice 2004;18:325–40.

18. Hosoya M, Kobayaski R, Ishii T, et al. Vocal hygiene education program reduces surgical interventions for benign vocal fold lesions: a randomized controlled trial. Laryngoscope 2018;128(11):2593–9.

19. Johns M. Update on the etiology, diagnosis, and treatment of vocal fold nodules, polyps, and cysts. Curr Opin Otolaryngol Head Neck Surg 2003;11: 456–61.

20. Hartnick C, Ballif C, DeGuzman V, et al. Indirect vs direct voice therpay for children with vocal nodules: a randomized clinical trial. JAMA Otolaryngol Head Neck Surg 2018;144(2):156–63.

21. Schindler A, Mozzanica F, Ginocchio D, et al. Vocal improvement after voice therapy in the treatment of benign vocal fold lesions. Acta Otorhinolaryngol Ital 2012; 32(5):304–8.

22. Yiu E, Lo M, Barrett E. A systematic review of resonant voice therapy. Int J Speech Lang Pathol 2017;19:17–29.

23. Angadi V, Croake D, Stemple J. Effects of vocal function exercises: a systematic review. J Voice 2019;33(1):124.e13-34.

24. Ribeiro VV, Pedrosa V, Silverio KCA, et al. Laryngeal manual therapies for behavioral dysphonia: a systematic review and meta-analysis. J Voice 2018;32(5): 553–63.
25. De Bodt M, Patteeuw T, Versele A. Temporal variables in voice therapy. J Voice 2015;29:611–7.
26. Chen M, Cheng L, Li C, et al. Nonsurgical treatment for vocal fold leukoplakia: an analysis of 178 cases. Biomed Res Int 2017;2017:6958250.

Diagnosis and Treatment of Benign Pediatric Lesions

Tiffiny A. Hron, MD[a], Katherine R. Kavanagh, MD[b,c], Nicole Murray, MD[b,c],*

KEYWORDS

- Dysphonia • Vocal nodule • Vocal fold polyp • Vocal fold cyst
- Vocal fold granuloma • Post-cricoid vascular cushion

KEY POINTS

- Dysphonia is prevalent in pediatrics, and the impact of dysphonia on children is variable.
- Pediatric dysphonia should be pursued to rule out a potentially dangerous pathology, such as laryngeal obstruction.
- Dysphonia must be evaluated by laryngeal examination with flexible laryngoscopy, flexible or rigid videostroboscopy, or microlaryngoscopy, if awake techniques are not feasible.
- Vocal nodules are the most common benign vocal lesions in pediatrics; other diagnoses, such as vocal fold polyps, cysts, granulomas, sulcus vocalis, and vascular anomalies, are less frequently identified.
- Given the variability of the impact on children, physicians should tailor treatment to match individual patients and, therefore, be an advocate for the pediatric patient.

 Video content accompanies this article at http://www.oto.theclinics.com.

IMPORTANCE OF DYSPHONIA IN PEDIATRICS

Dysphonia is estimated to affect up to 30% of people in their lifetimes.[1] Prevalence in childhood is difficult to pin down, and studies vary in some interesting ways. A frequently quoted 1975 study showed childhood prevalence to be 24%, but most newer and larger studies reveal smaller numbers.[2] Dysphonia was found in 4% of pre-schoolers (n = 2445) and 6% of 8 year olds (n = 7389) when screened by expert speech pathologists.[3,4] When 7-year-old to 16-year-old students were screened by

All authors have nothing to disclose.
[a] Harvard Medical School, Tufts University School of Medicine, Massachusetts General Hospital, Center for Laryngeal Surgery & Voice Rehabilitation, One Bowdoin Sq, 11th Floor, Boston, MA 02114, USA; [b] Pediatric Otolaryngology, Connecticut Children's Medical Center, 282 Washington, 2L, Hartford, CT 06106, USA; [c] Department of Otolaryngology-Head and Neck Surgery, University of Connecticut Medical School, Farmington, CT, USA
* Corresponding author. Pediatric Otolaryngology, Connecticut Children's Medical Center, 282 Washington, 2L, Hartford, CT 06106, USA
E-mail address: lnmurray@connecticutchildrens.org

speech pathologists plus stroboscopy, benign vocal lesions with hoarseness were found in 17% (n = 617).[5] The most ambitious prevalence study involved screening more than 60 million children with parental questionnaires and this revealed a prevalence of only 1.4%.[6] These variations suggest that parents may not be the most reliable reporters of voice health. This was demonstrated in the speech pathologist screening study previously mentioned, where 5% of all children who "never had a voice problem" were found to have dysphonia when formally assessed.[4]

The impact of the voice on a patient guides the treatment of voice disorders—the size of the lesion is much less important than whether or not the patients' vocal needs are met. The impact of dysphonia in pediatrics is variable. Sometimes there is no effect on a child, even when the parents are bothered a great deal, or there can be significant and underappreciated psychosocial impairments. Dysphonic children are perceived more negatively by peers[7] and adults,[8] and studies also have shown a striking potential quality-of-life detriment: hoarse toddlers can struggle with behavioral problems and older children can believe that their voice makes them inadequate.[9]

CLINICAL PRESENTATION AND DIAGNOSIS IN PEDIATRICS

Dysphonia or aphonia in a newborn usually triggers an evaluation prior to discharge. Dysphonia in a child, however, commonly has an insidious onset and may be missed for months or years, as parents become slowly accustomed to the voice.[4] A survey of pediatricians found that only 17% routinely assess children for voice problems.[10] Dysphonia thus often is recognized in a school setting or at a routine physician visit when a teacher, school-based speech and language pathologist, or health care provider hears the voice in conversation. Medical attention for dysphonia may be delayed in all age groups, but children are particularly at risk for this.

Dysphonia in an infant or child should be evaluated with laryngoscopy for 2 main reasons. First and foremost, the dysphonia may herald a life-threatening condition. Congenital laryngeal paresis may be the first sign of a Chiari malformation or a cardiac malformation. Respiratory papillomatosis must be treated before airway compromise ensues. Second, as discussed previously, dysphonia can have significant impact on the quality of life of a child. The American Academy of Otolaryngology–Head and Neck Surgery published guidelines for dysphonia in 2018 that echoed these concerns.[11] So when a hoarse infant or child presents to otolaryngology, 3 things must be done:

1. Rule out potentially dangerous disease processes.
2. Make a proper diagnosis.
3. Intervene as appropriate.

History and Physical

History

Specific elements of a voice history include details of the voice complaint: quality, volume, projection, fatigue, and loss as well as vocal pain or strain. Aphonia is of special concern because it may indicate impending airway compromise or severe abnormalities, such as extensive papillomatosis or glottic foreign body. The time frame should be noted, including sudden onset versus gradual onset, constant or intermittent difficulty, and stable versus worsening voice. Birth history, any intubations, and any surgeries of the chest or neck are relevant. Dysphonia must be distinguished from hypernasality and dysarthria. A voice review of systems includes swallow and airway symptoms, cough, throat clearing, seasonal allergies, lung diseases like asthma, and thyroid disorders. Lastly, the nature of voice use should be elicited, including the identification of patients with heavy voice use, such as singers, athletes, performers, and vocal overdoers.

Impact

A voice history is not complete without assessment of impact. There are many useful validated adult and pediatric voice impact self-assessments.[12–14] Most pediatric questionnaires are designed to be answered by the parent as proxy, because this is how nearly all information is gathered in pediatrics. In laryngology, however, this is problematic because parents have been shown to overestimate the impact of their child's voice disorder (or under-recognize the presence of dysphonia, as discussed previously), more so in younger children.[15] Accurate assessment of impact, from the child's point of view, is critical: this drives motivation to comply with diagnostic as well as therapeutic interventions, and compliance is the ultimate determinant of success of any voice intervention in a child. If differences between parental concerns and the child's concerns are encountered, this provides a rich opportunity to discuss intervention options, timing, and the overall risk/benefit ratio, especially where benign vocal lesions are concerned.

Physical

It is important to listen and characterize the voice and compare this to the perception of the concerned party as well as perception of the patient. A convenient auditory–perceptual analysis can be recorded using the grade, roughness, breathiness, asthenia, and strain (GRBAS) scale, in which each component gets a score of 0, 1, 2, or 3 for normal, slight, moderate, or severe abnormality, respectively. The voice characteristics may guide an otolaryngologist toward a diagnosis. For example, a breathy dysphonia may be more likely to result from glottic insufficiency, such as incomplete closure secondary to mass effect.[16–18] A voice-related examination also includes noting surgical scars or other trauma, neck abnormalities, oral and oropharyngeal abnormalities, stridor or stertor, strap muscle tenderness, neuromuscular issues, thyrohyoid narrowing/pain, posture, nasality, and breath support.

Laryngoscopy

The next step in the work-up is a careful visual examination of the larynx. In pediatrics, this is the most difficult portion of the examination but must be performed. In infants and younger children, awake transnasal flexible laryngoscopy is used most frequently. This may require bracing or restraint in very young children. Typically, older children are able to participate willingly when a clinician is well armed with developmentally appropriate techniques. Flexible nasopharyngoscopes are available in sizes as small as 2.4-mm diameter, which can fit easily into the newborn nose, which has a width of approximately 3 mm.[19] The passing of a laryngoscope causes no more than mild and temporary discomfort in infants and young children, and it provides good visualization of vocal fold movement and morphology. The examination can be done in newborns with generally only mild vital sign changes.[20]

High-resolution distal-chip flexible laryngoscopes provide enhanced image quality and definition to the laryngeal examination and are useful particularly in assessing and distinguishing benign pathology. Videostroboscopy provides assessment of laryngeal vibration and glottic closure. Although videostroboscopy can be performed with a standard flexible laryngoscope, there is a significant benefit when it is performed with either a high-resolution distal-chip laryngoscope or a rigid transoral laryngoscope. Flexible distal-chip stroboscopy has been shown successful even in very young children.[21] Rigid videostroboscopy also can be performed in children, with several large studies showing success in 2 year olds to 16 year olds.[5,22,23] Demirci and colleagues[23] queried 35 patients, ages 7 to 15, who underwent both transnasal and transoral videostroboscopy and 80% preferred the transoral examination to avoid nasal pain and irritation. The remainder preferred transnasal examination due to gagging.

The goal of laryngoscopy is to get a good exam in order to make an accurate diagnosis, and whether it is performed transnasally or transorally depends on the method that works best for the specific patient in the hands of a given clinician. Flexible laryngoscopy is the mainstay for most otolaryngologists caring for young patients, but it can miss subtle pathology. The addition of videostroboscopy to flexible laryngoscopy has been shown in studies to change the diagnosis in 47% of adults[24] and 34% of children.[25]

To improve patient tolerance of any type of laryngoscopy, the authors use a variety of techniques, matched to age and degree of patient buy-in. Younger children are encouraged to be brave and are promised a toy of their choice as a reward. For transnasal stroboscopy, seeing their "boogers" is remarked as kind of funny; for transoral stroboscopy, the scope is likened to a toothbrush at their tonsils. Voice exercises that are done during laryngoscopy are practiced beforehand. With older children, bravery is still encouraged but also empowering them as partners is attempted. Honesty is paramount—a false promise of no discomfort is counterproductive. The optimal goal is the long game, which is patient and parent buy-in to the entire process of diagnosis and treatment. If a clinician can learn what bothers a child about the voice and engages the child in diagnosis, the clinician can improve the child's engagement in treatment, which is paramount for children with benign vocal lesions.

If no form of awake laryngoscopy can be done, then other methods are required. Some physicians have found mild sedation to be useful.[22] Laryngeal ultrasound has been studied as an option particularly in the setting of vocal fold paresis,[26] but it cannot yet distinguish papilloma from nodules, and this is a significant limitation.[27] If a patient is simply unable to tolerate any form of awake laryngoscopy, then operative suspension microlaryngoscopy can be considered. Functional characteristics cannot be assessed under anesthesia, but laryngeal anatomy can; a diagnosis is found in most cases.

PATHOLOGY

Vocal nodules are the most common cause of dysphonia in children in all studies; rates vary between 48% and 96%.[2,5,28–30] So although it is important to remember that not all children with dysphonia have nodules, the data confirm that many do. The authors, therefore, focus on the diagnosis and treatment of nodules and then finally discuss the diagnosis and treatment of the remaining benign vocal lesions in children, which are cysts, polyps, sulcus vocalis, and benign neoplasms, including vascular lesions. Other causes of dysphonia in children that must not be disregarded, and are discussed elsewhere in this issue, include vocal fold palsy, respiratory papillomatosis, functional disorders, and malignant neoplasms.

Vocal Nodules

Nodules typically are firm bilateral lesions located along the mid-medial edge of the membranous vocal folds (**Fig. 1**). Children with nodules present with a rough or strained voice that develops over time. Alternately, a history of recurrent voice loss with increasingly poor recovery is obtained. Nodules are the result of phonotrauma: the vibrational stress of heavy use leads to the development of firm fibrovascular tissue between the epithelium and superficial lamina propria.[31] The natural history of

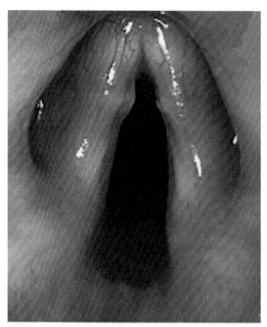

Fig. 1. Operative laryngoscopy of a nondysphonic child who underwent triple endoscopy for chronic cough and croup. Note bilateral vocal fold nodules, which are asymptomatic.

nodules in children remains controversial, due to the nature of vocal fold development and the difficulty in visualization with appropriate magnification and clarity. A 2007 study sought to characterize whether or not nodules diagnosed in childhood persist into adolescence. It showed that 21% of adolescents in this cohort still had dysphonia, with persistent nodules representing 29% of the group (47% in teenage girls).[32]

Treatment of vocal nodules

Treatment in children of all benign vocal fold lesions (eg, nodules, cysts, and polyps) is guided by their vocal needs—just as it is in adults. The otolaryngologist, speech pathologist, and parent must work together as a team to determine the appropriate degree of intervention in each situation. Intervention must be tailored not only to the pathology but also to a child's ability to participate with diagnostic and treatment regimens, and, lastly, to the impact on the child. As an advocate for the child, the otolaryngologist also must remember that parental reports of voice impact do not always correlate to a child's report[15]; treatment decisions should include impact and buy-in from the child's point of view, whenever possible. Due to the wide variability in disease impact, the decision to treat nodules, and dysphonia in general, is individualized.

There are 2 critical questions in children: (1) Is the child failing to meet their needs? and (2) Is the child able to cooperate with treatment? If the answer to either question is no, then no intervention or therapy need be considered. The impact question is best determined by child self-assessment: is the child bothered by the sound of the voice? Alternately, is the child's engagement with peers or participation in school impaired by the voice? Is the child being teased? The cooperation question must be explored based on developmental status and motivation for improvement. The child who is bothered by the voice has motivation to change it, whereas the child who is not bothered, no matter how bothered the parent is, likely is not motivated to comply with voice hygiene or cessation of vocally abusive behaviors.

Voice therapy for nodules

The primary treatment modality for children with nodules is voice therapy. A speech pathologist performs a voice assessment and develops a treatment plan. Although there are no formal age criteria for therapy to be successful, a child must have the maturity to cooperate and apply the techniques; children over 3 years of age can be evaluated for stimulability for therapy. When properly selected, speech therapy is highly successful in children.[33] Tezcaner and colleagues[34] reported improvement in all subjective and objective voice measures after therapy in 39 children ages 7 to 14; success was attributed to teamwork with parents and teachers to change vocally abusive behaviors.

Phonomicrosurgery for nodules

Phonomicrosurgery in children generally is avoided for several reasons. First, there are limitations in equipment as related to patient size: the laryngoscope must be large enough to provide precise visualization while allowing room for bimanual microsurgical instrumentation and simultaneous ventilation. Second, a child needs to follow strict postoperative recommendations, including voice rest, speech therapy, and laryngoscopy. Third, and perhaps most important, humans are not born with a fully developed larynx. Neonates are devoid of the layered microstructure found in the adult larynx, and this develops over time.[35] The length of the vocal fold increases with age.[36,37] What the impact of surgery is on the developing larynx is not known. Fourth, most benign vocal lesions in children improve or resolve without surgery.

Phonomicrosurgery for benign vocal lesions in children thus often is considered a last resort. In experienced centers, phonomicrosurgery on children can be performed following the same principles as in the adult population. The ideal candidate is a mature child who is significantly impacted, who has shown compliance with laryngoscopy and voice therapy techniques, and who is highly motivated for improvement. Outcomes studies for surgery for pediatric nodules, specifically, are limited to older questionnaire-only studies; they show potential voice improvement but underscore the sentiments regarding meticulous risk-benefit consideration and patient selection.[38–40]

Other Benign Vocal Lesions

Vocal fold polyps

Vocal fold polyps are sessile or pedunculated masses of the midmembranous vocal fold. They typically are unilateral. When filled with blood, they are called hemorrhagic polyps. These are uncommon but present in children.[5] Like vocal fold nodules, they are phonotraumatic lesions, but, unlike vocal fold nodules, they typically occur from episodes of intense phonotrauma or from a single vocally abusive event, such as screaming at a concert. They often are associated with phase asymmetry on stroboscopy. Treatment options in children are limited to no treatment, if a child is not impacted or is not a surgical candidate, versus phonomicrosurgery. Although voice therapy is not effective in adults, it may prove useful in children to prevent recurrence caused by persistent vocal abuse.

Vocal fold cysts

Vocal fold cysts are categorized as mucoid or epidermoid in nature. Mucoid cysts are believed to arise from an obstructed duct in the superficial lamina propria. Epidermoid cysts are less common and are believed the result of congenital cell rests or injured mucosa that gets under the epithelium. When subepithelial, vocal fold cysts typically are found along the medial edge of the membranous vocal folds. When intracordal, the vocal fold cysts can be found embedded in the superficial lamina propria or attached to the vocal ligament (**Fig. 2**).

As with vocal fold polyps, phonomicrosurgery is considered for most vocal fold cysts because speech therapy alone does not achieve adequate improvement in voice. There are significant challenges with resection of vocal fold cysts compared with polyps. Vocal fold cysts may be associated with other anomalies, such as a sulcus deformity or mucosal bridge. These can be challenging to diagnose during office laryngoscopy, so meticulous inspection under high-power magnification must be done in the operating room before surgical resection. A subepithelial saline infusion into the superficial lamina propria can aid in the detection of these.[41] Cysts must be removed in their entirety to avoid recurrence. This can be more difficult with mucoid cysts, given their fragility. Intracordal cysts can be the most difficult, because they require careful dissection within the superficial lamina propria to minimize injury to normal tissue. Additionally, intracordal cysts replace a substantial portion of the superficial lamina propria such that even with careful microdissection, removal leaves a deficit that does not regenerate and cannot be replaced. Therefore, careful consideration must be given to the risk-benefit ratio for removal of these lesions.

Vocal fold granulomas

Vocal fold granulomas are inflammatory lesions of the larynx that typically occur at an area of mucosal disruption. Most often they are associated with mechanical trauma from intubation,[42] but other causative factors include any repetitive mucosal disruption, such as chronic cough, throat clearing, vocal tics, or even a surgically created defect (**Fig. 3**, Video 1). Vocal fold granulomas are located most often at the vocal process of the arytenoids, where they may have a bilobed appearance. The thin overlying mucosa at the vocal process predisposes to perichondrial disruption, inflammation, and granulation tissue, and this can be further exacerbated by reflux and vocal hyperfunction.

Vocal fold granulomas primarily are treated conservatively and aggressively by (1) minimizing hyperfunction with speech therapy and (2) preventing further inflammation

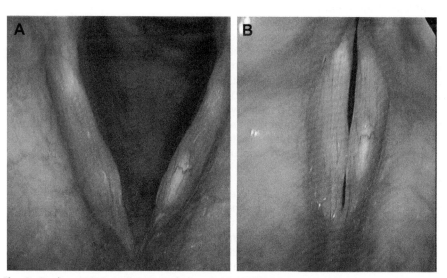

Fig. 2. Stroboscopic examination of the glottis. Bilateral intracordal cyst are noted in a 22 year old with presenting with dysphonia for the last several years.

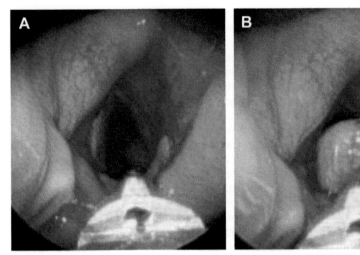

Fig. 3. Operative laryngoscopy during inspiration (*A*) and expiration (*B*) of a right vocal fold granuloma in a 2-year-old child with prolonged intubation. There was immediate respiratory distress and aphonia on extubation attempts. This granuloma was removed easily with optical forceps and did not recur. Video available online.

with reflux therapy. The lateral cricoarytenoid is most responsible for the hyperfunction that propagates inflammation at the vocal process by causing a hyper-rotation of the arytenoids.[43] More aggressive treatments are considered when conservative management fails or when the granuloma causes glottal obstruction. Although resection alone comes with a high recurrence rate, this can be minimized by continuing speech therapy and antireflux therapy. Botulinum toxin injection into the lateral cricoarytenoid muscle can be used as an adjunct in adults to decrease hyperfunction of this muscle. The risks of hypophonia, dysphagia, and aspiration, and the difficulty of injecting a child in clinic, make this a less attractive option in children.

Vocal fold ectasias and varices

Vocal fold ectasias and varices are vascular anomalies of the subepithelium. Varices typically are tortuous vessels whereas ectasias are discrete vascular malformations. Hochman and colleagues[44] observed that these lesions occurred most often at the superolateral limit of propagation of the mucosal wave and hypothesized that a whiplash effect of the vasculature is created as the mucosal wave abruptly changes direction. Because varices and ectasias rupture more easily than normal-appearing vessels, they are of concern in patients with recurrent vocal fold hemorrhage. It is uncommon to find a pediatric patient with repetitive vocal fold hemorrhage, and, therefore, these often do not necessitate treatment in children. They do, however, provide important evidence to a patient's vocal use pattern.

Sulcus vocalis

Sulcus vocalis occurs when vocal fold epithelium adheres to the vocal ligament or muscle. It may be associated with other pathology, such as cysts and mucosal bridges. The etiology is unclear but both congenital and acquired origins have been proposed.[45,46] Diagnosis can be challenging, particularly in pediatrics, when good visualization in the office can be difficult (**Fig. 4**). In the operating room, diagnosis can be aided with a subepithelial saline infusion into the superficial lamina propria. Unfortunately, no treatments are effective, so management primarily consists of providing prognostic information.

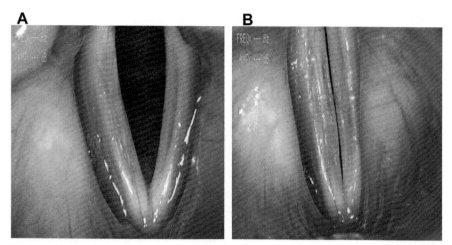

Fig. 4. Stroboscopic examination of the glottis. Bilateral sulcus vocalis in a 16-year-old high school student involved in musical theater.

Vascular Lesions

Hemangiomas

Glottic and subglottic hemangiomas can have an impact on the airway and present more often with stridor than with dysphonia. These lesions generally present as recurrent croup in young infants, which responds to steroids but then recurs. Confirmation of the diagnosis may require laryngoscopy in the operating room; in some cases, a subglottic lesion is visible on awake flexible laryngoscopy. Larger transglottic lesions may be diagnosed easily on awake scope. Systemic propranolol is the treatment of choice and works well on most lesions. Airway hemangiomas were reviewed recently by Darrow.[47]

Postcricoid vascular anomalies/cushions

Postcricoid vascular anomalies/cushion lesions are proliferations of vasculature in the postcricoid area that can appear as a grape-like spherical mass that becomes prominent during straining. These lesions present in infants as stridor or dysphagia more than dysphonia, and they often are referred to as a "disappearing lesion": they are visible on awake laryngoscopy but often cannot be identified under anesthesia unless specific Valsalva or Trendelenburg maneuvers are used. This pathology is encountered only rarely in the adult population. Hoff and Koltai[48] merged anatomic and clinical data to show that there is a normal postcricoid venous plexus in infancy that regresses, and that, if looking at this region in normal infants during crying, postcricoid swelling during expiration often is seen. Large lesions may cause significant esophageal or airway obstruction and seem to be properly considered venous malformations.[49,50] Small lesions may be observed clinically; symptomatic lesions may be treated successfully with endoscopic laser ablation.[51]

SUMMARY

Dysphonia in infants and children is common and should be evaluated with laryngoscopy for proper and safe management. Benign vocal lesions, specifically nodules, are the most common cause. Intervention, whether behavioral or surgical, should be considered only in a child who is both highly motivated for improvement and developmentally able to comply with therapy; otherwise, time and health care dollars are wasted. Voice therapy is highly successful. Phonomicrosurgery in children is technically challenging but can be performed by experienced surgeons in carefully chosen children. Further research is needed regarding outcomes in pediatric phonomicrosurgery.

SUPPLEMENTARY DATA

Supplementary data related to this article can be found online at https://doi.org/10.1016/j.otc.2019.03.010.

REFERENCES

1. Roy N, Merrill RM, Gray SD, et al. Voice disorders in the general 485 population: prevalence, risk factors, and occupational impact. Laryngoscope 2005;115: 1988–95.
2. Silverman EM. Incidence of chronic hoarseness among school-age children. J Speech Hear Disord 1975;40:211–5.
3. Duff MC, Proctor A, Yairi E. Prevalence of voice disorders in African American and European American preschoolers. J Voice 2004;18:348–53.
4. Carding PN, Roulstone S, Northstone K, et al. The prevalence of childhood dysphonia: a cross-sectional study. J Voice 2006;20:623–30.
5. Akif Kiliç M, Okur E, Yildirim I, et al. The prevalence of vocal fold nodules in school age children. Int J Pediatr Otorhinolaryngol 2004;68:409–12.
6. Bhattacharyya N. The prevalence of pediatric voice and swallowing problems in the United States. Laryngoscope 2015;125:746–50.
7. Lass NJ, Ruscello DM, Stout LL, et al. Peer perceptions of normal and voice-disordered children. Folia Phoniatr (Basel) 1991;43:29–35.
8. Ruscello DM, Lass NJ, Podbesek J. Listeners' perceptions of normal and voice-disordered children. Folia Phoniatr (Basel) 1988;40:290–6.
9. Connor NP, Cohen SB, Theis SM, et al. Attitudes of children with dysphonia. J Voice 2008;22:197–209.
10. Sajisevi M, Cohen S, Raynor E. Pediatrician approach to dysphonia. Int J Pediatr Otorhinolaryngol 2014;18:1365–7.
11. Stachler RJ, Francis DO, Schwartz SR, et al. Clinical practice guideline: hoarseness (dysphonia) (update). Otolaryngol Head Neck Surg 2018;158:S1–42.
12. Jacobson B, Johnson A, Grywalsky C. The voice handicap index (VHI): development and validation. Am J Speech Lang Pathol 1997;6:66–70.
13. Boseley ME, Cunningham MJ, Volk MS, et al. Validation of the pediatric voice-related quality-of-life survey. Arch Otolaryngol Head Neck Surg 2006;132: 717–20.
14. Zur KB, Cotton S, Kelchner L, et al. Pediatric Voice Handicap Index (pVHI): a new tool for evaluating pediatric dysphonia. Int J Pediatr Otorhinolaryngol 2007;71: 77–82.
15. Cohen W, Wynne DM. Parent and child responses to the pediatric voice-related Quality-of-Life Questionnaire. J Voice 2015;29:299–303.
16. Hirano M. Clinical examination of the voice. New York: Springer Verlag; 1981. p. 81–4.
17. Dejonckere PH, Wieneke GH. GRBAS-scaling of pathological voices: reliability, clinical relevance and differentiated correlation with acoustical measurements, especially with cepstral measurements. Proceedings of the 22nd IALP Congress. Hannover, Germany, August 10-14, 1992.

18. De Bodt MS, Wuyts FL, Van de Heyning PH, et al. Test–retest study of the GRBAS scale: influence of experience and professional background on perceptual rating of voice quality. J Voice 1997;11:74–80.

19. Contencin P, Gumpert L, Sleiman J, et al. Nasal fossae dimensions in the neonate and young infant: a computed tomographic scan study. Arch Otolaryngol Head Neck Surg 1999;125:777–81.

20. Ongkasuwan J, Yung KC, Courey MS. The physiologic impact of transnasal flexible endoscopy. Laryngoscope 2012;122:1331–4.

21. Hartnick CJ, Zeitels SM. Pediatric video laryngo-stroboscopy. Int J Pediatr Otorhinolaryngol 2005;69:215–9.

22. Mackiewicz-Nartowicz H, Sinkiewicz A, Bielecka A. Laryngovideostroboscopy in children–diagnostic possibilities and constraints. Int J Pediatr Otorhinolaryngol 2011;75:1015–7.

23. Demirci S, Tuzuner A, Callioglu EE, et al. Rigid or flexible laryngoscope: the preference of children. Int J Pediatr Otorhinolaryngol 2015;79:1330–2.

24. Sataloff RT, Spiegel JR, Hawkshaw MJ. Strobovideolaryngoscopy: results and clinical value. Ann Otol Rhinol Laryngol 1991;100:725–7.

25. Mortensen M, Schaberg M, Woo P. Diagnostic contributions of videolaryngostroboscopy in the pediatric population. Arch Otolaryngol Head Neck Surg 2010;136: 75–9.

26. Ongkasuwan J, Ocampo E, Tran B. Laryngeal ultrasound and vocal fold movement in the pediatric cardiovascular intensive care unit. Laryngoscope 2017; 127:167–72.

27. Ongkasuwan J, Devore D, Hollas S, et al. Laryngeal ultrasound and pediatric vocal fold nodules. Laryngoscope 2017;127:676–8.

28. Wynne DM, Cohen W. The Pediatric voice clinic: our experience of 81 children referred over 28 months. Clin Otolaryngol 2012;37:318–20.

29. Papsin BC, Pengilly AJ, Leighton SEJ. The developing role of a pediatric voice clinic: a review of our experience. J Laryngol Otol 1996;110:1022–6.

30. Smith M. Care of the child's voice: a pediatric otolaryngologists perspective. Semin Speech Lang 2013;34:63–70.

31. Gray SD, Hammond E, Hanson DF. Benign pathologic responses of the larynx. Ann Otol Rhinol Laryngol 1995;104:13–8.

32. De Bodt MS, Ketelslangers K, Peeters T, et al. Evolution of vocal nodules from childhood to adolescence. J Voice 2007;21:151–6.

33. Ongkasuwan J, Friedman EM. Is voice therapy effective in the management of vocal fold nodules in children? Laryngoscope 2013;123:2930–1.

34. Tezcaner CZ, Ozgursoy SK, Dursun G. Changes after voice therapy in objective and subjective voice measurements of pediatric patients with vocal nodules. Eur Arch Otorhinolaryngol 2009;266:1923–7.

35. Ishii K, Yamashita K, Akita M, et al. Age-related development of the arrangement of the connective tissue fibers in the lamina propria of the human vocal fold. Ann Otol Rhinol Laryngol 2000;109:1055–64.

36. Hirano M, Kurita S, Nakashima T. Growth, development, and aging of human vocal folds. In: Abbs J, editor. Vocal fold physiology. San Diego (CA): College Hill Press; 1983. p. 23–43.

37. Hartnick CJ, Rehbar R, Prasad V. Development and maturation of the pediatric human vocal fold lamina propria. Laryngoscope 2005;115:4–15.

38. Benjamin B, Croxson G. Vocal nodules in children. Ann Otol Rhinol Laryngol 1987;96:530–3.

39. Kay NJ. Vocal nodules in children–aetiology and management. J Laryngol Otol 1982;96:731–6.
40. Mori K. Vocal fold nodules in children: preferable therapy. Int J Pediatr Otorhinolaryngol 1999;49(Suppl 1):S303–6.
41. Burns JA, Friedman AD, Lutch MJ, et al. Subepithelial vocal fold infusion: a useful diagnostic and therapeutic technique. Ann Otol Rhinol Laryngol 2012;121:224–30.
42. Jang M, Basa K, Levi J. Risk factors for laryngeal trauma and granuloma formation in pediatric intubations. Int J Pediatr Otorhinolaryngol 2018;107:45–52.
43. Zeitels SM. Atlas of phonomicrosurgery and other endolaryngeal procedures for benign and malignant disease. San Diego (CA): Singular Thomson Learning; 2001.
44. Hochman I, Sataloff RT, Hillman RE, et al. Ectasias and varices of the vocal fold: clearing the striking zone. Ann Otol Rhinol Laryngol 1999;108:10–6.
45. Giovanni A, Chanteret C, Lagier A. Sulcus vocalis: a review. Eur Arch Otorhinolaryngol 2007;264:337–44.
46. Bouchayer M, Cornut G, Witzig E. Epidermoid cysts, sulci, and mucosal bridges of the true vocal cord: a report of 157 cases. Laryngoscope 1985;95:1087–94.
47. Darrow DH. Management of infantile hemangiomas of the airway. Otolaryngol Clin North Am 2018;51:133–46.
48. Hoff SR, Koltai PJ. The "postcricoid cushion:" observations on the vascular anatomy of the posterior cricoid region. Arch Otolaryngol Head Neck Surg 2012;138:562–71.
49. Parhizkar N, Manning SC, Inglis AF, et al. How airway venous malformations differ from airway infantile hemangiomas. Arch Otolaryngol Head Neck Surg 2011;137:352–7.
50. Roehm C, Chelius DC, Larrier D, et al. Postcricoid vascular lesions: histopathological and immunohistochemical diagnosis. Laryngoscope 2011;121:397–403.
51. Zur KB, Wood RE, Elluru RG. Pediatric postcricoid vascular malformation: a diagnostic and treatment challenge. Int J Pediatr Otorhinolaryngol 2005;69:1697–701.

Update on Recurrent Respiratory Papillomatosis

Craig S. Derkay, MD[a],*, Andrew E. Bluher, MD[b]

KEYWORDS

- Recurrent respiratory papillomas (RRP) • Human papillomavirus (HPV)
- HPV vaccine • Bevacizumab

KEY POINTS

- Recurrent respiratory papillomatosis (RRP) is a devastating, albeit rare, disease in which papillomas of the airway cause hoarseness and airway obstruction.
- Surgical therapy for RRP requires a team approach with otolaryngologists, anesthesia providers, and operating room personnel working together in a facility properly equipped to manage difficult airways.
- The recent introduction of a 9-valent human papillomavirus vaccine offers hope for prevention of transmission of the virus to neonates and may significantly reduce the future incidence of RRP and oropharyngeal cancers.
- There has been a decline in RRP incidence in Australia following the implementation of a national vaccination program, with some evidence that this decline is also occurring in the United States and Canada.
- Systemic bevacizumab treatment seems to be effective in severe uncontrolled disease.

INTRODUCTION

Recurrent respiratory papillomatosis (RRP) remains a challenging disease afflicting children and adults alike, resulting in an estimated $120 million per year in United States healthcare–related costs, with annual costs per patient approaching $60,000.[1] In addition, it is associated with higher rates of depression and voice-related quality of life.[2] Although the prevalence of RRP has declined since the introduction of the human papillomavirus (HPV) vaccine 12 years ago, RRP remains the most common benign laryngeal neoplasm in children. RRP is unique in its high rate

---

Disclosure: The authors have nothing to disclose.

[a] Department of Otolaryngology–Head and Neck Surgery, Pediatric Otolaryngology, Eastern Virginia Medical School, Children's Hospital of the King's Daughters, 601 Children's Lane, 2nd Floor, Norfolk, VA 23507, USA; [b] Department of Otolaryngology–Head and Neck Surgery, Eastern Virginia Medical School, Sentara Norfolk General Hospital, 600 Gresham Drive, Suite 1100, Norfolk, VA 23507, USA
* Corresponding author.
E-mail address: craig.derkay@chkd.org

Otolaryngol Clin N Am 52 (2019) 669–679
https://doi.org/10.1016/j.otc.2019.03.011
0030-6665/19/© 2019 Elsevier Inc. All rights reserved.

of multisite recurrence, its high burden on patient quality of life, and its high associated healthcare costs. This article summarizes recent advances in the understanding of the natural history and quality-of-life burden of RRP as a disease, as well as basic science advancements in prevention and treatment, giving hope for a future with lower prevalence of RRP and improved treatment options.

NATURAL HISTORY AND RISK FACTORS

RRP is a heterogeneous disease, caused by 2 primary strains of HPV (HPV 6 and HPV 11), and presenting in 2 predominant age groups (juvenile onset, occurring before the age of 12 years; and adult onset, occurring from 20–40 years of age). It has previously been shown that HPV 11 is the more aggressive viral strain of the two, and that younger age of presentation is associated with a more detrimental course.[3]

Recent work has brought an understanding of the natural history of adult-onset RRP closer. Benedict and colleagues[4] described a cohort of 83 previously untreated patients with adult-onset RRP and noted that the membranous vocal folds are most frequently involved. They also noted a significant association between involvement of subglottic and posterior glottic regions and proton pump inhibitor usage, prompting further questions on the potential interplay between laryngopharyngeal reflux, its medical therapies, and RRP.

Formánek and colleagues[5] further explored the association between laryngopharyngeal reflux and RRP, examining biopsied tissue from 20 RRP-afflicted individuals as well as 20 controls for evidence of pepsin within the tissue, as well as the presence herpes simplex virus type 2 (HSV-2). They found that 40% of patients with RRP had pepsin within biopsied tissue and 45% had HSV-2, whereas controls had neither. This finding suggests that inflammatory and immunosuppressive effects of laryngopharyngeal reflux and HSV may trigger or exacerbate papillomatous growth. Further study is indicated regarding whether treatment of these concomitant conditions could assist in adult RRP management.

Epidemiology

RRP is a disease of viral cause characterized by the proliferation of benign squamous papilloma within the aerodigestive tract (**Fig. 1**). RRP is both the most common benign

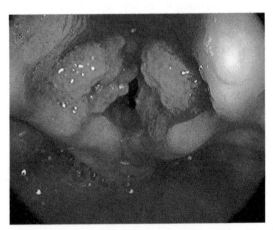

Fig. 1. Direct laryngoscopic view of pediatric larynx afflicted by RRP. Benign squamous epithelial proliferation is appreciable along laryngeal surface of epiglottis, bilateral aryepiglottic folds, false vocal folds, and true vocal folds.

neoplasm of the larynx among children and the second most frequent cause of childhood hoarseness.[6,7] The disease is often difficult to treat because of its tendency to recur and spread throughout the aerodigestive tract. Although it most often involves the larynx, RRP may involve the entire aerodigestive tract. The course of the disease is variable; some patients experience spontaneous remission, whereas others may develop aggressive papillomatous growth and respiratory compromise that requires multiple surgical procedures through many years in addition to the emotional burden to the patients and their families associated with the need for repeated surgery.[8]

The true incidence and prevalence of RRP are uncertain. Numerous studies have been performed to elucidate the true incidence of RRP. It has been estimated that between 80 and 1500 new cases of childhood-onset RRP occur in the United States each year,[9–11] although the introduction of the HPV vaccine seems to be drastically decreasing the number of new cases in the United States and abroad.[12]

Prevention

The potential exists for a breakthrough in prevention of RRP with the emergence of widespread use of the 9-valent HPV vaccine (Gardasil; Merck) in the developed world. The vaccine has been used for the prevention of cervical cancer, adenocarcinoma in situ, and intraepithelial neoplasia grades 1 through 3; vulvar and vaginal intraepithelial neoplasia grades 2 and 3; and genital warts associated with HPVs 6, 11, 16, and 18.[13–15] It seems that the vaccine is most effective if administered to individuals who have not yet become sexually active.

Accordingly, the Centers for Disease Control and Prevention (CDC) Advisory Committee on Immunization Practices has recommended that all boys and girls 11 to 12 years of age (before the age of sexual debut) be vaccinated.[16,17] The original quadrivalent HPV (qHPV) vaccine has been replaced with a 9-valent vaccine.[18] The quadrivalent vaccine is no longer being manufactured and the CDC currently does not recommend revaccinating those who originally received the quadrivalent vaccine. The HPV vaccine was developed similar to the hepatitis B vaccine in that it contains viruslike particles (VLPs). VLP vaccines contain repetitive high-density displays of viral surface proteins, which present conformational viral epitopes that can elicit strong T-cell and B-cell immune responses. In addition, because the VLPs lack genetic material, they provide a safer alternative to attenuated viruses. However, they are not designed to have any effect on the episomal state of established epithelial infections, although there is substantial cross reactivity.

Perhaps the most promising result of the past 2 years has been the publication of a 5-year report from Australia following the implementation of a systematic HPV vaccination program.[12] The quadrivalent vaccine was introduced in 2007 with greater than 80% uptake in girls and greater than 75% uptake in boys of at least 2 doses. A decline in RRP annual incidence was found from 0.16 to 0.02 per 100,000 children with only 15 incident cases noted nationwide; none of the mothers of these children were vaccinated. This study constitutes the first demonstration that the HPV vaccine may hold promise in the eradication of RRP. Ongoing surveillance studies in the United States and Canada are attempting to document similar declines despite lower levels of population uptake.

Limitations of Vaccination Programs

Vaccination holds a great deal of promise for a vast reduction in RRP incidence; however, it is limited by suboptimal rates of acceptance among providers and patient families in countries such as the United States. According to the 2016 National Immunization Survey, although 91% of teens aged 13 to 17 years report having received 1 or more doses of the hepatitis B vaccine and 82% received the meningo-coccal conjugate vaccine, only 60% received a single dose of the HPV vaccine.[19] There is continued debate regarding how to improve vaccination acceptance rates. Nwanodi and colleagues[20] found that adding audiovisual aids as well as a patient health education handout increased both HPV-specific knowledge and vaccination acceptance rates.

Several obstacles have limited universal vaccination, including moral objections and cost. Critics have objected that vaccination programs may promote unprotected and dangerous sexual activity, concerns that have not been supported by the scientific literature regarding acquired immunodeficiency syndrome awareness and contracep-tion. Public health officials may have justifiable concerns about the merits of HPV vaccination based on the financial and logistic burdens that may be imposed on fam-ilies and schools, and they also may legitimately worry about adverse events that might occur with large-scale vaccination programs that involve children. The cost to fully immunize all 11-year-old and 12-year-old girls and boys is estimated to exceed $1.7 billion per year, although this expense will be offset by a predicted decrease of $6.5 billion in healthcare costs annually.[21]

Vaccination as Treatment Adjuvant

The vaccine's efficacy as a therapeutic option is markedly more limited,[22,23] and although the antibody response may be boosted by administration, surveillance for future lesions should be continued. Somewhat surprisingly, there is increasing evi-dence that the vaccine may be beneficial in treatment of patients with existing disease in reducing regrowth after debridement. At a minimum, it is likely to prevent infection from other HPV subtypes and protect recipients against oral, anal, penile, and cervical cancer from the oncogenic strains covered in the vaccine.

Young and colleagues[24] reported on a retrospective cohort of 20 patients who received qHPV vaccine as part of their treatments and found a significant increase in intersurgical intervals. Male patients seemed to get more benefit than female pa-tients and 13 of 20 patients experienced complete or partial responses. A recent case report highlights the potential benefit of vaccination for the patients with RRP already afflicted with HPV. A 2-year-old child with RRP was treated with 3 doses of 9-valent HPV vaccine, and subsequently experienced an increase in average intersur-gical interval from 46 days to 340 days.[25]

Dion and colleagues[26] performed a systematic review of adjuvant HPV vaccination and found decreases in disease recurrence disease burden or increased intersurgical intervals in 9 of 12 studies and those with active disease. These improvements may be explained by Tjon Pian Gi and colleagues'[27] findings of increased mean HPV-specific antibody reactivity in 6 patients with RRP after vaccine administration. They showed a mean antibody reactivity increasing from 1125 mean fluorescence intensity (MFI) to 4690 MFI ($P<.001$) and 3-fold improvements in intersurgical intervals. This potential for use of the vaccine as treatment may extend well beyond childhood. In a proof-of-concept effort, Makiyama and colleagues[28] showed a significant increase in anti-body titers in adult male patients with RRP aged 32 to 74 years after vaccination with q-HPV vaccine. Kin Cho Goon[29] also reported on a cohort of 12 adult patients with RRP aged 27 to 78 years who experienced a greater than 7-fold decrease in their incidence rates of papillomatosis requiring surgical intervention after receiving vacci-nation with qHPV.[29]

The RRP Task Force is prospectively gathering information from its membership on the HPV vaccination of children with existing disease to better understand the benefit of vaccination in patients less than 9 years of age.

Classic Surgical Management

At present, there is no cure for RRP, and no single modality has consistently been shown to be effective in the eradication of RRP. The current standard of care is surgical therapy with a goal of complete removal of papilloma and preservation of normal structures. In patients in whom anterior or posterior commissure disease or highly aggressive papilloma are present, the goal may be subtotal removal with clearing of the airway. It is advisable to debulk as much disease as possible while preserving normal morphology and anatomy and preventing the complications of subglottic and glottic stenosis, web formation, and resulting airway stenosis. Even with the removal of all clinically evident papilloma, latent virus remains in adjacent tissue.

Adjuvant Treatment Modalities

Although surgical management remains the mainstay therapy for RRP, ultimately as many as 20% of patients with the disease require some form of adjuvant therapy.[30] The most widely adopted criteria for initiating adjuvant therapy are a requirement for more than 4 surgical procedures per year, rapid regrowth of papilloma disease with airway compromise, or distal multisite spread of disease.

Cidofovir

Multiple reports have stimulated interest in the intralesional injection of cidofovir for treatment of RRP. Cidofovir is a broad-spectrum antiviral agent, with virus toxicity affecting viruses beyond the Herpesviridae family. The US Food and Drug Administration (FDA) approved its use only for intravenous treatment of cytomegalovirus retinitis in patients with HIV. Despite being an off-label use per the FDA, and regardless of the lack of controlled, randomized, blinded clinical trials in children with RRP, cidofovir is currently the most frequently used adjuvant drug.[30,31] Pransky and colleagues[32] used this therapy in 10 children with severe RRP with short-term follow-up and showed a response in all 10 patients; long-term follow-up has been encouraging as well.[33,34] Similarly encouraging results have been reported by Naiman and colleagues[35,36] in a small cohort of adults and children treated with a protocol-driven approach using a high dose of cidofovir at 2-week intervals. Co and Woo[37] also showed efficacy in a small cohort of adults with RRP treated with serial office-based intralesional injections of cidofovir. In addition, encouraging successful treatments of pulmonary multicystic papillomatosis have used systemic and inhaled cidofovir.[38,39]

Based on animal studies that showed a high level of carcinogenicity, and based on case reports of progressive dysplasia in patients with RRP, guidelines have been published for clinicians interested in using cidofovir in their patients with RRP.[40,41] As a result, cidofovir is widely used off label for this disease in severely affected patients.[31] In a 10-year systematic review of the literature regarding RRP treated with intralesional cidofovir, complete resolution in 57% of all patients and partial response in 35% of patients were reported.[42] However, in the only existing double-blinded, randomized controlled study, which used what many consider to be a subtherapeutic dose of cidofovir, no statistical difference was seen between cidofovir and placebo in Derkay severity score, voice-handicap index, and a quality-of-life survey.[43] Reprogrammed RRP cells may provide a means to identify patients who are more likely to favorably respond to cidofovir or, for that matter, to other adjuvant drugs.[44]

A best-practice guideline based on the experience of 82 otolaryngologists describes specific indications for use of cidofovir.[31] Initiation of cidofovir is recommended in patients who require more than 6 surgeries per year, are experiencing decreasing intervals between surgery, or have extralaryngeal spread.

Recommendations are for a dose of less than 40 mg/kg in adults and less than 3 mg/kg in children. A therapeutic trial of a total of 5 injections at 2-week to 6- week intervals is recommended before abandoning this modality. Given the morbidity from multiple surgical interventions and the attendant risks of administering multiple general anesthetics, some clinicians have argued to begin the use of cidofovir early in the course of the disease in an effort to prevent future complications (Pransky, personal communication, RRP Task Force meeting, April 2018).

Bevacizumab

Bevacizumab (Avastin, Genentech, San Francisco, CA) is a recombinant monoclonal antibody to vascular endothelial growth factor (VEGF) that prevents its interaction with the VEGF receptor. First approved for use in the United States as a combination therapy for metastatic colon cancer, bevacizumab was developed with the aim of reducing neoplastic angiogenesis. It has since been approved for use in the treatment of a variety of neoplasms. Local intralesional injection has been used in RRP with some success. No detrimental vocal fold changes were observed on pathologic review of injected porcine laryngeal specimens.[45]

Systemic bevacizumab as a treatment of RRP has shown some dramatic successes in particularly severe cases refractory to other medical treatments.[46] Best and colleagues[47] found 8 patients nationwide with severe disease who were treated with 5 to 10 mg/kg every 2 to 4 weeks, with all showing at least a partial response. All patients have required continued treatment, with relapse noted when treatment intervals were extended too long; however, remission was achieved in select patients with intervals lengthened to 6 weeks.[48] A protocol for uniform treatment of severely affected patients with systemic bevacizumab is currently in development at Children's Hospital of Philadelphia and Johns Hopkins.[46,47] Current best-practice recommendations for systemic bevacizumab administration in the treatment of RRP include partnership with oncology services to do thorough off-label consent and arrange for infusions with hospital approval. The main monitored side effects are hypertension, thrombus formation, electrolyte imbalances, and renal damage. It is recommended to screen for the sequelae discussed earlier and obtain baseline studies including a cardiac echocardiogram. The patient's disease should first be debrided in the operating room, followed by bevacizumab 10 mg/kg intravenous infusion for 1.5 hours. The next procedure and infusion are performed in approximately 3 weeks to reexamine and debride as needed. As a response is observed, intervals for debridement and infusion intervals can be liberalized to 2 to 3 months. The duration of the infusion can be decreased as well. Patients without tracheal disease can be followed in clinic with flexible laryngoscopy. Because of a 28-day black box warning for performing surgical procedures while receiving bevacizumab, it is important to avoid open cases in this time period to reduce the risk of wound breakdown.

FRONTIERS IN MEDICAL TREATMENT

Until HPV vaccination rates reach levels high enough to promote herd immunity, RRP will still demand further advances in treatment. Although surgical treatment continues to be vital in both the diagnosis as well as control of the disease, major strides are being made in the basic sciences that may pave the way to further medical therapies. These advances range from novel DNA vaccine development to the investigational use of therapies previously used to treat viral hepatitis or ocular neoplastic disease. For instance, pegylated interferon, used in the treatment and cure of hepatitis C viral infection, was recently used in the treatment of a child with severe RRP with good response.[49]

Deoxyribonucleic Acid Vaccination

Although the quadrivalent HPV L1 vaccine shows promise in helping to control recurrent disease, Deoxyribonucleic acid (DNA) vaccines are under investigation for their greater potential therapeutic benefit. Preventive vaccines are composed primarily of inactivated viral proteins; in contrast, DNA vaccines contain the DNA blueprints to synthesize these proteins. DNA vaccines are harnessed by recipient cells to repeatedly transcribe these proteins, subsequently promoting a greater immune response than simply presenting those antigens during an isolated injection. In addition, DNA vaccines are customizable such that antigenic proteins can be linked to other proteins, such as calreticulin, that may further enhance immune responses. Ahn and colleagues[50] administered a calreticulin-linked DNA vaccine encoding the HPV 11 E6 and E7 genes to mice that had previously been inoculated with an HPV 11 E6E7-expressing tumor cell line, and found a specific HPV 11 CD-8–positive T-cell response as well as slowed tumor growth.

Programmed Death 1 and Programmed Death Ligand 1 Pathway Inhibitors

An additional promising line of research concerns programmed death 1 (PD-1) pathway inhibitors. The T-lymphocyte coinhibitory receptor and its ligand PD-L1 are thought to contribute to a locally immunosuppressed environment that allows immune system evasion and resultant papillomatous growth. Ahn and colleagues[50] reported increased rates of PD-1 T-lymphocyte infiltration and PD-L1 expression on both papilloma and infiltrating immune cells. Targeting the PD-1 pathway thus represents a promising strategy for treating RRP. A prospective clinical trial for treatment of adult RRP with an anti–PD-L1 antibody called avelumab (Bavencio) is currently underway at the National Institutes of Health.[51] A nonrandomized phase II trial for treatment of adults with tracheal, bronchial, pulmonary, or severe laryngeal RRP with the anti–PD-1 monoclonal antibody pembrolizumab (Keytruda) is currently undergoing FDA review.[52]

Registry and Task Force Initiatives

It should be stressed that participation in national and regional protocols of adjuvant treatment modalities is essential for the scientific community to learn more about RRP. Initially, a national registry of patients with RRP was performed through the cooperation of the American Society of Pediatric Otolaryngology (ASPO) and the CDC.[11] A second registry study was begun in 2016 with CDC support. Prospective data on incidence are being collected from 25 sites and a retrospective collection of cases from the same centers dating back 20 years is being totaled to assess at the effect of HPV vaccination on the incidence of juvenile-onset RRP (JORRP). The RRP Task Force, made up of the principal investigators at each of the registry sites as well as representatives from the adult RRP research community, patient/parent advocacy groups, and international RRP experts meets twice yearly to facilitate research initiatives.

Other Considerations

Until recently, data have been limited regarding voice outcomes for patients treated with each modality. A 2009 study reviewed voice outcomes in 2 cohorts of children with active JORRP.[53] One group was defined as the CO_2 laser cohort if more than 25% of their procedures were performed with the CO_2 laser; a second group was treated almost exclusively with the microdebrider. Outcome measures included measurements of jitter, shimmer, noise/harmonic ratio, and perceptive analysis by a trained speech-language pathologist. Scores were consistently lower in the microdebrider cohort, which indicates improved voice and suggests that voice quality deteriorated with increased usage of the CO_2 laser (**Fig. 2**). Larger cohorts, inclusion of adult

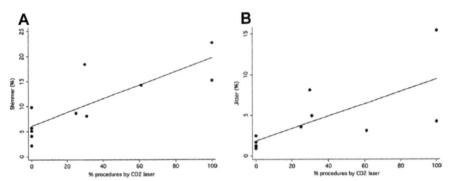

Fig. 2. Immediate postoperative (*A*) shimmer and (*B*) jitter acoustic score versus proportion of surgical procedures by CO_2 laser. Regression lines shown on scatter plot; shimmer Spearman correlation coefficient rho = 0.793; P = .004. Jitter Spearman correlation coefficient rho = 0.827; P = .002. (*Data from* Holler T, Allegro J, Chadha NK, et al. Voice outcomes following repeated surgical resection of laryngeal papillomata in children. Otolaryngol Head Neck Surg 2009;141(4):522–6.)

patients, and longer-term follow-up may be needed to make more generalized statements about the effects of a specific surgical modality on the voice.

Children with newly diagnosed RRP warrant a substantial time commitment on the part of their otolaryngologists to engage the families in a frank and open discussion of the disease and its management. Support groups such as the Recurrent Respiratory Papilloma Foundation (www.rrpf.org) can be a vital resource for information and support. A team-centered approach to the care of patients with RRP is optimal.

SUMMARY

RRP is a frustrating, capricious disease with the potential for morbid consequences because of its involvement of the airway and the risk of malignant degeneration. The goals of surgical therapy are to maintain a safe airway with a serviceable voice while avoiding excessive scarring. When children require surgical therapy more frequently than 4 times in 12 months or have evidence of distal spread of RRP outside of the larynx, adjuvant medical therapy should be considered.

Universal or near-universal use of an HPV vaccine that provides protection against HPVs 6 and 11 may do for RRP what the *Haemophilus influenzae* B vaccine has done for *H influenzae* type B epiglottitis: virtually eliminate new cases in less than a decade. Because of the recurrent nature of RRP and the potential for airway obstruction, parental support and education can be invaluable to the safety of children with RRP.

REFERENCES

1. Bishai D, Kashima H, Shah K. The cost of juvenile-onset recurrent respiratory papillomatosis. Arch Otolaryngol Head Neck Surg 2000;126(8):935–9.
2. San Giorgi MRM, Aaltonen LM, Rihkanen H, et al. Quality of life of patients with recurrent respiratory papillomatosis. Laryngoscope 2017;127(8):1826–31.
3. Gallagher TQ, Derkay CS. Recurrent respiratory papillomatosis: update 2008. Curr Opin Otolaryngol Head Neck Surg 2008;16(6):536–42.
4. Benedict PA, Ruiz R, Yoo M, et al. Laryngeal distribution of recurrent respiratory papillomatosis in a previously untreated cohort. Laryngoscope 2018;128(1): 138–43.

5. Formánek M, Jančatová D, Komínek P, et al. Laryngopharyngeal reflux and herpes simplex virus type 2 are possible risk factors for adult-onset recurrent respiratory papillomatosis (prospective case-control study). Clin Otolaryngol 2017; 42(3):597–601.

6. Mounts P, Shah KV, Kashima H. Viral etiology of juvenile- and adult-onset squamous papilloma of the larynx. Proc Natl Acad Sci U S A 1982;79:5425.

7. Morgan AH, Zitsch RP. Recurrent respiratory papillomatosis in children: a retrospective study of management and complications. Ear Nose Throat J 1986;65:19.

8. Lindman JP, Lewis LS, Accortt N, et al. Use of the pediatric quality of life inventory to assess the health-related quality of life in children with recurrent respiratory papillomatosis. Ann Otol Rhinol Laryngol 2005;114:499.

9. Derkay CS. Task force on recurrent respiratory papillomas. A preliminary report. Arch Otolaryngol Head Neck Surg 1995;121:1386.

10. Reeves WC, Ruparelia SS, Swanson KI, et al. National registry for juvenile-onset recurrent respiratory papillomatosis. Arch Otolaryngol Head Neck Surg 2003; 129:976.

11. Armstrong LR, Preston EJ, Reichert M, et al. Incidence and prevalence of recurrent respiratory papillomatosis among children in Atlanta and Seattle. Clin Infect Dis 2000;31:107.

12. Novakovic D, Cheng ATL, Zurynski Y, et al. A prospective study of the incidence of juvenile-onset recurrent respiratory papillomatosis after implementation of a National HPV Vaccination Program. J Infect Dis 2018;217(2):208–12.

13. Future II study group. Quadrivalent vaccine against HPV to prevent high-grade cervical lesions. N Engl J Med 2007;356:1915–27.

14. Tenti P, Zappatore R, Migliora P, et al. Perinatal transmission of human papillomavirus from gravidas with latent infections. Obstet Gynecol 1999;93:475.

15. Garland SM, Hernandez-Avila M, Wheeler CM, et al. Quadrivalent vaccine against human papillomavirus to prevent anogenital diseases. N Engl J Med 2007;356:1928–43.

16. Markowitz LE, Dunne EF, Saraiya M, et al. Quadrivalent HPV: recommendations of the ACIP. Available at: www.cdc.gov/nip/vaccine/hpv. Accessed March 23, 2007.

17. Markowitz LE, Dunne EF, Saraiya M, et al. Recommendations on the use of quadrivalent human papillomavirus vaccine in males—Advisory Committee on Immunization Practices (ACIP) 2011. Available at: www.cdc.gov/mmwr/preview/mmwrhtml/mm6050a3.htm. Accessed September 3, 2018.

18. Iversen OE, Miranda MJ, Ulied A, et al. Immunogenicity of the 9-valent HPV vaccine using 2-dose regimens in girls and boys vs a 3-dose regimen in women. JAMA 2016;316:2411.

19. Walker TY, Elam-Evans LD, Singleton JA, et al. National, regional, state, and selected local area vaccination coverage among adolescents aged 13-17 years - United States, 2016. MMWR Morb Mortal Wkly Rep 2017;66(33):874–82.

20. Nwanodi O, Salisbury H, Bay C. Multimodal counseling interventions: effect on human papilloma virus vaccination acceptance. Healthcare (Basel) 2017;5(4) [pii:E86].

21. Elbasha EH, Dasbach EJ, Insinga RP. Model for assessing human papillomavirus vaccination strategies. Emerg Infect Dis 2007;13(1):28–41.

22. Villa LL, Costa RL, Petta CA, et al. Prophylactic quadrivalent HPV (types 6, 11, 16 and 18) L1 virus-like particle vaccine in young women: a randomized double-blind placebo controlled multi-centre phase II efficacy trial. Lancet Oncol 2005; 6:271–8.

23. Markowitz LE. HPV vaccines prophylactic, not therapeutic. JAMA 2007;298(7): 805–6.

24. Young DL, Moore MM, Halstead LA. The use of the quadrivalent human papillomavirus vaccine (Gardasil) as adjuvant therapy in the treatment of recurrent respiratory papilloma. J Voice 2015;29:223.

25. Sullivan C, Curtis S, Mouzakes J. Therapeutic use of the HPV vaccine in recurrent respiratory papillomatosis: a case report. Int J Pediatr Otorhinolaryngol 2017;93: 103–6.

26. Dion GR, Teng S, Boyd LR, et al. Adjuvant human papillomavirus vaccination for secondary prevention: a systematic review. JAMA Otolaryngol Head Neck Surg 2017;143(6):614–22.

27. Tjon Pian Gi RE, San Giorgi MR, Pawlita M, et al. Immunological response to quadrivalent HPV vaccine in treatment of recurrent respiratory papillomatosis. Eur Arch Otorhinolaryngol 2016;273:3231.

28. Makiyama K, Hirai R, Matsuzaki H. Gardasil vaccination for recurrent laryngeal papillomatosis in adult men: first report: changes in HPV antibody titer. J Voice 2017;31(1):104–6.

29. Kin Cho Goon P, Scholtz LU, Sudhoff H. Recurrent respiratory papillomatosis (RRP)-time for a reckoning? Laryngoscope Investig Otolaryngol 2017;2(4):184–6.

30. Schraff S, Derkay CS, Burke B, et al. American Society of Pediatric Otolaryngology members' experience with recurrent respiratory papillomatosis and the use of adjuvant therapy. Arch Otolaryngol Head Neck Surg 2004;130:1039.

31. Derkay CS, Volsky PG, Rosen CA, et al. Current use of intralesional cidofovir for recurrent respiratory papillomatosis. Laryngoscope 2013;123(3):705–12.

32. Pransky SM, Magit AE, Kearns DB, et al. Intralesional cidofovir for recurrent respiratory papillomatosis in children. Arch Otolaryngol Head Neck Surg 1999;125: 1143.

33. Pransky SM, Albright JT, Magit AE. Long-term follow-up of pediatric recurrent respiratory papillomatosis managed with intralesional cidofovir. Laryngoscope 2003; 113:1583.

34. Pransky SM, Brewster DF, Magit AE, et al. Clinical update on 10 children treated with intralesional cidofovir injections for severe recurrent respiratory papillomatosis. Arch Otolaryngol Head Neck Surg 2000;126:1239.

35. Naiman AN, Ayari S, Nicollas R, et al. Intermediate-term and long-term results after treatment by cidofovir and excision in juvenile laryngeal papillomatosis. Ann Otol Rhinol Laryngol 2006;115:667.

36. Naiman AN, Ceruse P, Coulombeau B, et al. Intralesional cidofovir and surgical excision for laryngeal papillomatosis. Laryngoscope 2003;113:2174.

37. Co J, Woo P. Serial office-based intralesional injection of cidofovir in adult-onset recurrent respiratory papillomatosis. Ann Otol Rhinol Laryngol 2004;113:859.

38. Dancey DR, Chamberlain DW, Krajden M, et al. Successful treatment of juvenile laryngeal papillomatosis-related multicystic lung disease with cidofovir: case report and review of the literature. Chest 2000;118:1210.

39. Ksiazek J, Prager JD, Sun GH, et al. Inhaled cidofovir as an adjuvant therapy for recurrent respiratory papillomatosis. Otolaryngol Head Neck Surg 2011;144(4): 639–41.

40. Wemer RD, Lee JH, Hoffman HT, et al. Case of progressive dysplasia concomitant with intralesional cidofovir administration for recurrent respiratory papillomatosis. Ann Otol Rhinol Laryngol 2005;114:836.

41. Derkay C. Cidofovir for recurrent respiratory papillomatosis (RRP): a reassessment of risks. Int J Pediatr Otorhinolaryngol 2005;69:1465.

42. Chadha NK, James A. Adjuvant antiviral therapy for recurrent respiratory papillomatosis. Cochrane Database Syst Rev 2010;(1):CD005053.
43. McMurray JS, Connor N, Ford CN. Cidofovir efficacy in recurrent respiratory papillomatosis: a randomized, double-blind, placebo-controlled study. Ann Otol Rhinol Laryngol 2008;117(7):477–83.
44. Yuan H, Myers S, Wang J, et al. Use of reprogrammed cells to identify therapy for respiratory papillomatosis. N Engl J Med 2012;367(13):1220–7.
45. Ahmed MM, Connor MP, Palazzolo M, et al. Effect of high-dose vocal fold injection of cidofovir and bevacizumab in a porcine model. Laryngoscope 2017; 127(3):671–5.
46. Zur KB, Fox E. Bevacizumab chemotherapy for management of pulmonary and laryngotracheal papillomatosis in a child. Laryngoscope 2017;127(7):1538–42.
47. Best SR, Mohr M, Zur KB. Systemic bevacizumab for recurrent respiratory papillomatosis: a national survey. Laryngoscope 2017;127(10):2225–9.
48. Bedoya A, Glisinski K, Clarke J, et al. Systemic bevacizumab for recurrent respiratory papillomatosis: a single center experience of two cases. Am J Case Rep 2017;18:842–6.
49. Maunsell R, Bellomo-Brandão MA. Pegylated interferon for treating severe recurrent respiratory papillomatosis in a child: case report. Sao Paulo Med J 2017; 136(4):376–81.
50. Ahn J, Bishop JA, Roden RBS, et al. The PD-1 and PD-L1 pathway in recurrent respiratory papillomatosis. Laryngoscope 2018;128(1):E27–32.
51. Hinrichs CS. Avelumab for people with recurrent respiratory papillomatosis. 2018. Available at: Clinicaltrials.gov. Accessed September 3, 2018.
52. Pai S. Pembrolizumab for HPV-associated recurrent respiratory papilloma patients with laryngeal, tracheal and/or pulmonary involvement. 2018. Available at: Clinicaltrials.gov. Accessed September 3, 2018.
53. Holler T, Allegro J, Chadha NK, et al. Voice outcomes following repeated surgical resection of laryngeal papillomata in children. Otolaryngol Head Neck Surg 2009; 141(4):522–6.

Unilateral Vocal Fold Immobility in Children

M. Elise Graham, MD, FRCSC[a],*, Marshall E. Smith, MD[b,c]

KEYWORDS

- Unilateral vocal fold immobility • Dysphonia • Recurrent laryngeal nerve injury

KEY POINTS

- Unilateral vocal fold paralysis is a common complication of many procedures of the neck and chest, but is particularly common following cardiothoracic surgery.
- Symptoms of unilateral vocal fold immobility are related to all functions of the larynx, and may include stridor, dysphonia, and dysphagia.
- Work-up of these patients should include imaging of the entire length of the recurrent laryngeal nerve for anatomic causes, if the cause is not clear from patient history.
- Static and dynamic treatment options are available, depending on patient and family preference and local expertise.
- Treating unilateral vocal fold paralysis may improve voice, swallowing function, and quality of life.

INTRODUCTION

Unilateral vocal fold immobility, or unilateral vocal fold paralysis (UVFP), may lead to airway, swallowing, and vocal impairment in affected children. It is recognized as a major cause of dysphonia and dysphagia, and may cause stridor. Thus, it may affect each major component of laryngeal function. The course of the recurrent laryngeal nerve (RLN) puts it at risk for iatrogenic injury. There are various other described causes, and many cases are idiopathic.

Several terms are used synonymously with UVFP. Most descriptive may be impaired vocal fold mobility, which covers the spectrum of vocal fold dysfunction. Vocal fold paresis implies reduced mobility but not complete immobility. Paralysis is a term theoretically reserved for complete lower motor nerve dysfunction, although

Disclosure: The authors have nothing to disclose.
[a] Department of Otolaryngology–Head and Neck Surgery, Children's Hospital at London Health Sciences Centre, Schulich School of Medicine, Western University, 800 Commissioner's Road East, London, Ontario N6A 5W9, Canada; [b] Division of Otolaryngology–Head and Neck Surgery, University of Utah, Salt Lake City, Utah, USA; [c] Division of Otolaryngology, University of Utah School of Medicine, 50 North Medical Drive, SOM 3C120, Salt Lake City, UT 84132, USA
* Corresponding author.
E-mail address: elise.graham@lhsc.on.ca

Otolaryngol Clin N Am 52 (2019) 681–692
https://doi.org/10.1016/j.otc.2019.03.012
0030-6665/19/© 2019 Elsevier Inc. All rights reserved.

oto.theclinics.com

complete flaccidity and denervation are not typically seen in vivo. It is suspected that, even in complete nerve transection, aberrant reinnervation or synkinesis leads to the variable presentations seen, from minimal dysfunction to profound dysphonia.[1]

This article describes the prevalence, causes, and treatment options for this common problem, and reviews treatment options, with an emphasis on the importance of recognizing and appropriately managing UVFP for best outcomes for affected children.

EPIDEMIOLOGY

It is difficult to obtain an accurate estimate of the prevalence of UVFP in children, although hundreds of cases of UVFP have been detailed in the literature. Diagnosis by conventional flexible nasolaryngoscopy (FNL) in children can be complicated by floppy supraglottic structures, suboptimal view, and secretions, making it challenging even for experienced examiners.[2] Techniques for diagnosis are improving with the ability to record and replay examinations and higher-definition equipment. These technological advances and improved infant survival rates may mean that the true incidence of UVFP is higher than what is currently reported, and should likely be reevaluated.

Some estimates place the number of cases seen in tertiary pediatric otolaryngologists' practices between 4 and 10 per year.[3] Vocal fold paralysis (VFP), either unilateral or bilateral, represents 10% of all congenital laryngeal lesions, second only to laryngomalacia in frequency as a cause of neonatal stridor.[4,5] Unilateral paralysis typically presents before 24 months of age, with many patients presenting before the age of 1 year.[6,7] In a 10-year series by Daya and colleagues,[7] 65% of patients presenting before 1 year were symptomatic at birth. There is no gender predilection for UVFP.[8] The volume of cardiac surgery performed at an institution also has an impact on the frequency of UVFP seen.

CAUSES

UVFP is a physical finding, not a diagnosis. In cases in which a UVFP is identified, the cause of the paralysis must be elucidated. Similar causes of UVFP exist for both adults and children, although the frequencies of each cause are not the same. Certain insults may cause UVFP but are more commonly associated with bilateral VFP, and these are not addressed in this article. Common causes of bilateral VFP include Arnold-Chiari and other central malformations, many peripheral neuropathies such as myasthenia gravis, and inflammatory and infectious causes such as Guillain-Barré syndrome and varicella infection.[7,9,10] Vincristine toxicity is also most commonly a cause of bilateral VFP but has been reported to cause UVFP[11,12] (**Box 1**).

Traumatic Causes

Iatrogenic causes of UVFP are by far the most common.[7,13] The left RLN is particularly at risk for injury during surgery because it descends into the chest, loops below the arch of the aorta, and returns superiorly to enter the larynx at the cricothyroid joint.

Cardiothoracic surgeries are most commonly implicated in RLN injury and resultant paralysis.[9,14] In a meta-analysis including more than 5600 infants following cardiothoracic surgery, nearly 10% were found to have UVFP.[15] However, in those studies in which all patients underwent routine laryngoscopy after cardiothoracic surgery, the proportion with UVFP was much higher, at 30%, compared with patients who showed symptoms. Patent ductus arteriosus (PDA) repair has a particularly high risk of injury to the left RLN.[15-17] A prospective study of all infants in a single institution revealed that

> **Box 1**
> **Recognized causes for unilateral vocal fold paralysis in children**
>
> Surgery/iatrogenic
>   Cardiac surgery (especially patent ductus arteriosus ligation)
>   Tracheoesophageal fistula/esophageal atresia repair
>   Branchial anomaly excision
>   Thyroidectomy
>   Intubation
>   Extracorporeal membrane oxygenation or central venous catheter placement
>
> Trauma
>
> Cardiovascular anomalies
>
> Neoplasia
>
> Idiopathic

nearly one-quarter of preterm infants and those with very low weight at the time of surgery (<1250 g) sustained nerve injury.[17] Laryngeal symptoms such as dysphonia and stridor were not apparent in 14% of the study infants, and injuries again might have been missed without prospective endoscopy. Although some patients compensate well for this injury, others might dysfunction that is not recognized until school age. The authors suggest that all infants undergoing cardiothoracic surgery, and particularly those who are very small or preterm, should be evaluated postoperatively by an experienced otolaryngologist with a flexible laryngoscopy.

Repair of esophageal atresia (EA) with or without associated tracheoesophageal fistula (TEF) can result in UVFP or bilateral VFP, with an incidence as high as 22% in some studies.[18–21] Although concurrent airway lesions are common in patients with EA/TEF, recent work suggests that unilateral VFP is more likely a consequence of repair rather than of the anomaly itself.[19]

Any procedure involving structures with a proximate anatomic relationship to the RLN places children at risk for UVFP. The RLN lies in the tracheoesophageal groove posterior to the thyroid and is intimately related to the gland anatomically. As such, thyroidectomy is a well-described cause of UVFP in adults, and estimates of the rate of UVFP in children after this procedure range from 1% to 6%.[22–24] Branchial anomalies likewise have a defined relationship with the RLN, particularly the more rare third and fourth branchial anomalies.[25,26] There are also reports of right RLN injury resulting from extracorporeal membrane oxygenation cannulation and resection of giant cervicofacial teratomas in neonates.[27,28]

Intubation with an inappropriately large or cuffed endotracheal tube can result in UVFP in adults.[29,30] UVFP from prolonged intubation in children has been reported, but less commonly.[8] Appropriate tube size and minimizing the duration of intubation are important to reduce the likelihood of this complication, in addition to the morbidity of subglottic stenosis.

Birth trauma is another recognized cause for both UVFP and bilateral VFP.[7,9,31–33] A systematic review and pooled analysis suggested birth trauma was more than twice as likely to lead to UVFP compared with idiopathic congenital vocal paralysis, which was more commonly bilateral.[31]

Idiopathic Causes

Idiopathic UVFP is the second largest etiologic category for UVFP after cardiothoracic surgery.[7,8] It is estimated to account for 36% to 47% of causes in a variety of series.[14,18,32] The pathophysiology may represent a viral neuropathy similar to Bell palsy or sudden sensorineural hearing loss, but this remains difficult to prove definitively.

Neoplastic Causes

Neoplasia is a less frequently described cause of UVFP in the pediatric population. Neoplasms involving the skull base, neck, or mediastinum can each result in UVFP. In the case of neoplasia, a slow, progressive process would be expected, initially affecting 1 side. Examples include benign and malignant thyroid neoplasms.

Cardiovascular Anomalies

Congenital cardiovascular anomalies frequently cause VFP, with the left RLN being more vulnerable to injury because of its longer course and proximity to the heart. Tetralogy of Fallot, ventricular septal defects, and cardiomegaly have all been associated with UVFP. Likewise, anomalies of the great vessels, including vascular rings, double aortic arch, and PDA, have all been implicated in vocal fold dysfunction.[5] Dilatation of the pulmonary artery can cause compression of the RLN, leading to the cardiovocal Ortner syndrome of infants.[34–37]

PRESENTATION

Patients with UVFP may be asymptomatic or have significant functional impairment. Any or all of the functions of the larynx may be affected. Three-quarters of affected children present with stridor.[6,7] Half experience dysphonia, and one-quarter have dysphagia. Other presentations may include poor cough, aspiration, recurrent pneumonias, reactive airway disease, and subtle feeding difficulties. Although patients with bilateral VFP may have a relatively normal voice and are more likely to present with respiratory distress, those with UVFP more frequently have hoarseness, breathiness, reduced vocal volume, or an abnormal cry.[38]

DIAGNOSTIC EVALUATION

The first step in evaluating a child with suspected UVFP is a thorough history and physical examination. Each facet of laryngeal function should be addressed. Is there stridor? What is the character of the child's voice or cry? Are there associated feeding difficulties? Recurrent pneumonias or aspiration might also indicate laryngeal disorder. Surgical history with focus on cardiothoracic surgery or any procedures of the neck and chest; past medical history of congenital anomalies; and birth history, including birth trauma, should be elucidated. Initial physical examination should focus on evidence of respiratory difficulty, including respiratory rate, intercostal in-drawing and retractions, and listening to the character of the child's voice. **Fig. 1** details the process for children in whom UVFP is suspected.

Flexible laryngoscopy in awake patients is the current gold standard for assessing vocal fold mobility. It provides a dynamic view of the larynx and supraglottic structures. In UVFP, depending on the time since injury, a flaccid, immobile, and possibly atrophic ipsilateral vocal fold might be visualized. The arytenoid might be anteriorly displaced or medially rotated, with loss of adduction on that side.[39] Most children can be diagnosed accurately with this method alone.[38] FNL provides a dynamic view with minimal distortion, is safe, and is fairly well tolerated. However, it is does have challenges, particularly in very young infants. Difficulty in visualization of the larynx by laryngoscopy is reported in up to 20% of patients less than 3 years of age.[40] Barriers include rapid respiratory rate, floppy supraglottic structures, secretions,

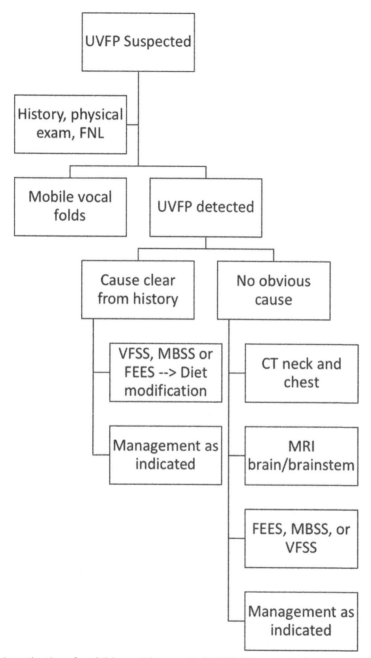

Fig. 1. Investigations for children with suspected UVFP. CT, computed tomography; VFSS, videofluoroscopic swallow study; MBSS, modified barium swallow study; FEES, functional endoscopic evaluation of swallowing. Management options are detailed in the text.

anterior positioning of the larynx, and a narrowed epiglottis. Clinicians appropriately use the quality of the cry and the clinical history as clues when the view is suboptimal; in the absence of sound or a clinical history, intrarater and inter-rater reliability of flexible laryngoscopy is only moderate.[2]

Because of these difficulties, many other methods have been proposed to evaluate the neonatal larynx for UVFP. Laryngeal ultrasonography is a promising method to evaluate the neonatal larynx. Recent work in the pediatric cardiovascular intensive care unit compared laryngeal ultrasonography with FNL, with the goal of preventing noxious stimuli to infants sensitive to subtle physiologic changes.[41] Although imperfect, the agreement between these two methods was substantial. Laryngeal ultrasonography may serve as a useful adjunct or replacement for FNL in certain situations.[42] Other proposed methods for evaluating pediatric patients for UVFP include audiometric measures, pulmonary function tests, and direct laryngoscopy under general anesthesia.[5,38,43–45] For various reasons, these methods have not as yet proved suitable replacements for laryngoscopy but may also be adjunctive. For example, the use of general anesthesia to assess vocal fold function might result in distortion of the larynx through poor placement of the laryngoscope blade or altered movement based on depth of anesthesia, leading to misdiagnosis of UVFP.[38,45,46] This potential pitfall can be circumvented with FNL before the administration of general anesthesia when a child is undergoing comprehensive airway evaluation in the operating room.

Once UVFP has been identified, subsequent work-up should focus on identification of the cause and determining functional impact on the affected child. If the cause is not clear from a suggestive past medical or surgical history, imaging is suggested to identify anatomic insults. Imaging should assess the length of the RLN and vagus nerve. The brain, brainstem, and skull base are best studied with MRI, and the neck and chest are better characterized using computed tomography (CT).

Swallow studies such as videofluoroscopic swallowing studies (VFSS) or modified barium swallow studies (MBSS) identify functional impairment and help direct dietary interventions to reduce the morbidity from possible aspiration. An alternative means to evaluate the safety of swallowing is a functional endoscopic evaluation of swallowing (FEES). In this examination, a flexible laryngoscope is introduced transnasally as multiple food consistencies are consumed, assessing for penetration or aspiration. FEES does not expose patients to radiation, and can also be used to test laryngeal sensation. However, it is slightly more invasive to patients, and there is a brief whiteout period during the swallow during which the bolus cannot be seen.

There is a role for operative bronchoscopy for the evaluation of the airway in children with UVFP when no other cause is identified in a noninvasive work-up and when the patient has additional airway symptoms. Up to 45% of patients with UVFP have synchronous lesions such as subglottic stenosis, cricoarytenoid joint fixation, or intubation granuloma.[7] A complete evaluation in the operating room is not necessarily indicated for patients with an obvious cause of VFP, such as following a PDA ligation.

Laryngeal electromyography (L-EMG) can be used to confirm UVFP in difficult cases. L-EMG can be performed on awake adults but requires general anesthesia in children (**Fig. 2**). This test assesses for the presence and morphology of motor unit action potentials (MUAPs) in the denervated muscles. The data regarding pediatric L-EMG are variable, with older publications suggesting that its clinical utility in predicting return of vocal function is limited.[47–51] Protocols and follow-up regimes vary across studies. A multi-institutional trial suggested that absence of MUAPs 6 months after injury from PDA ligation predicts a lower likelihood of functional recovery.[52] This finding may empower clinicians to intervene earlier to prevent the morbidity associated with UVFP rather than waiting many years hoping that the UVFP resolves. Normal MUAPs in the context of a persistently immobile vocal fold are also possible, and the interpretation of this scenario is more difficult.

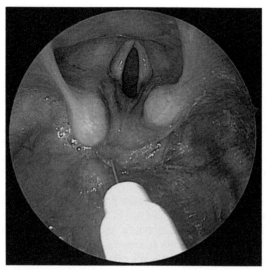

Fig. 2. Laryngeal electromyography. Electrode is seen inserted into the left posterior cricoarytenoid muscle.

MANAGEMENT
Importance of Treatment

UVFP caused by a transection of the RLN is unlikely to recover. After PDA ligation, a systematic review of the literature reported recovery rates ranging from zero to 33%.[53] Rates of recovery in UVFP caused by other factors also vary, with idiopathic causes recovering in roughly 40% of cases.[54] Even recovery is poorly defined, and there may not be neuromotor recovery despite an improved voice over time.

There are limited data to support the belief that children with persistent isolated UVFP will adjust without morbidity. Although some patients do not have significant dysfunction, it is not always possible to predict whether a relatively asymptomatic infant will have difficulty at school with vocal weakness. Premature, medically fragile children are disproportionately likely to sustain RLN injury after PDA ligation, and are less likely to recover.[17,54] A review of 120 infants following PDA ligation showed that nearly all those with UVFP were less than 1150 g[17] Those of a comparable weight without UVFP were discharged from hospital sooner and were significantly less likely to have a feeding tube at the time of discharge. Premature infants with UVFP following PDA ligation have long-term sequelae as well, with an increased incidence of bronchopulmonary dysplasia, reactive airway disease, and need for gastrostomy tube.[55] Patients with confirmed UVFP should be followed by a pediatric otolaryngologist at regular intervals and offered treatment to improve their function and quality of life.

Treatment Modalities

Speech therapy is advocated to be the first line in treatment of UVFP despite limited studies proving its efficacy in pediatric patients.[45,56] However, it may be helpful and is unlikely to cause harm. Adults benefit from speech/voice therapy. This cohort typically presents with recent onset of paralysis versus long-standing issues from infancy. Furthermore, age and maturity enable better compliance with recommendations in the adult patients.[57,58]

Injection medialization laryngoplasty (IML) is a mainstay of treatment of UVFP (**Fig. 3**). Polytetrafluoroethylene (Teflon) was an early permanent agent, but is now no longer used because of concerns regarding long-term effects, potential for granuloma formation, and irreversibility.[56] There are 3 reported cases of Teflon injection in pediatric patients.[33,59] All currently available agents are temporary, with varying durations of action. Options with experience and demonstrated efficacy in pediatric UVFP include Gelfoam, collagen, carboxymethylcellulose gel (Prolaryn Gel, Merz USA), and micronized acellular dermal matrix (Cymetra, Allergan USA).[56,59–61] IML has several advantages, including its ease, immediate effect, and temporary nature. A systematic review showed most patients had improved speech, swallowing, and aspiration after IML.[62] Need for repeated injection, judgment regarding degree of augmentation, and potentially unfavorable viscoelastic properties of the vocal fold following injection are pitfalls of the IML technique.[63]

Thyroplasty is less commonly used in pediatric patients, although it remains a common intervention in adults. The largest series in the literature reviewed 8 pediatric patients and found improvement in dysphagia and aspiration.[64] A recent systematic review only found 12 pediatric patients across 5 studies that were suitable for inclusion in its thyroplasty group.[62] Thyroplasty is still offered by a subset of pediatric otolaryngologists, usually in postpubertal patients complaining of aspiration, in whom other procedures are not suitable.[65] Arytenoid adduction is of theoretic utility to close larger posterior glottic gaps, but the laryngeal framework of very young children precludes its use in this population, because the arytenoid muscular process is less well defined and palpable. It may be used in adolescents with a large posterior glottic gap.[66]

A recent survey of trends in the management of UVFP by pediatric otolaryngologists showed that more than 20% would offer ansa cervicalis–RLN reinnervation procedures as a first-line therapy.[65] Comfort with this procedure and knowledge of its efficacy in pediatric patients is likely driving the shift toward reinnervation. The goal of laryngeal reinnervation is to provide bulk and tone to the denervated vocal fold, thereby allowing complete glottic closure from the contralateral vocal fold. It does not restore mobility. In adult populations, younger patients tended to have better voice outcomes from laryngeal reinnervation compared with thyroplasty.[67] Investigations

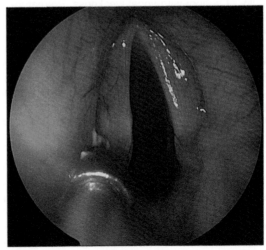

Fig. 3. Injection medialization laryngoplasty. Injection of temporary filler (in this case, micronized acellular dermal matrix) into the left vocal fold.

then extended into younger populations, first showing improved perceptual vocal outcomes in adolescents and young adults,[66] and then children less than 10 years old.[68] When ansa-RLN reinnervation is compared directly with IML, both interventions offer improvement in vocal function and vocal handicap scores.[39] However, long-term results and level of satisfaction were higher in the reinnervation group.

Studies show that reinnervation continues to improve vocal outcomes many years following RLN injury, with improved outcomes in patients with earlier intervention.[39,69] However, all patients seem to show benefit, independent of age. Swallowing outcomes have been less frequently evaluated in early investigations of reinnervation, but parental reports of dysphagia are improved postprocedure.[68] Reinnervation resulted in resolution of aspiration on barium swallow in a group of pediatric patients with UVFP, now expanding its indications beyond dysphonia.[70]

Reinnervation is a permanent intervention that does not alter the viscoelastic properties of the vocal fold through the introduction of a foreign body. There is no requirement for clinician judgment about degree of augmentation as in thyroplasty or IML. It does not affect laryngeal development or framework, and does not require an awake, cooperative patient. However, it does subject patients to an external incision. Reinnervation typically takes 4 to 6 months for evidence of effect, therefore the authors and many others perform concomitant IML with a resorbable implant to temporarily provide bulk and improve closure during the healing process. Continued improvement over time is noted up to 20 months postprocedure.[39]

REFERENCES

1. Crumley RL. Laryngeal synkinesis revisited. Ann Otol Rhinol Laryngol 2000;109: 365–71.
2. Liu YC, McElwee T, Musso M, et al. The reliability of flexible nasolaryngoscopy in the identification of vocal fold movement impairment in young infants. Int J Pediatr Otorhinolaryngol 2017;100:157–9.
3. Setlur J, Hartnick CJ. Management of unilateral true vocal cord paralysis in children. Curr Opin Otolaryngol Head Neck Surg 2012;20:497–501.
4. Holinger PH, Brown WT. Congenital webs, cysts, laryngoceles and other anomalies of the larynx. Ann Otol Rhinol Laryngol 1967;76:744–52.
5. Dedo DD. Pediatric vocal cord paralysis. Laryngoscope 1979;89:1378–84.
6. King EF, Blumin JH. Vocal cord paralysis in children. Curr Opin Otolaryngol Head Neck Surg 2009;17:483–7.
7. Daya H, Hosni A, Bejar-Solar I, et al. Pediatric vocal fold paralysis: a long-term retrospective study. Arch Otolaryngol Head Neck Surg 2000;126:21–5.
8. Tibbetts KM, Wu D, Hsu JV, et al. Etiology and long-term functional swallow outcomes in pediatric unilateral vocal fold immobility. Int J Pediatr Otorhinolaryngol 2016;88:179–83.
9. Gentile RD, Miller RH, Woodson GE. Vocal cord paralysis in children 1 year of age and younger. Ann Otol Rhinol Laryngol 1986;95:622–5.
10. Rizzardi E, Tagliaferro T, Snijders D, et al. Unilateral laryngeal paralysis in a newborn with congenital varicella syndrome. Int J Pediatr Otorhinolaryngol 2009;73:115–8.
11. Kuruvilla G, Perry S, Wilson B, et al. The natural history of vincristine-induced laryngeal paralysis in children. Arch Otolaryngol Head Neck Surg 2009;135: 101–5.
12. Annino DJ Jr, MacArthur CJ, Friedman EM. Vincristine-induced recurrent laryngeal nerve paralysis. Laryngoscope 1992;102:1260–2.

13. Zur KB. Vocal fold motion impairment. Curr Probl Pediatr Adolesc Health Care 2018;48:124–8.
14. Zbar RI, Smith RJ. Vocal fold paralysis in infants twelve months of age and younger. Otolaryngol Head Neck Surg 1996;114:18–21.
15. Strychowsky JE, Rukholm G, Gupta MK, et al. Unilateral vocal fold paralysis after congenital cardiothoracic surgery: a meta-analysis. Pediatrics 2014;133: e1708–23.
16. Zbar RI, Chen AH, Behrendt DM, et al. Incidence of vocal fold paralysis in infants undergoing ligation of patent ductus arteriosus. Ann Thorac Surg 1996;61:814–6.
17. Smith ME, King JD, Elsherif A, et al. Should all newborns who undergo patent ductus arteriosus ligation be examined for vocal fold mobility? Laryngoscope 2009;119:1606–9.
18. Cohen SR, Geller KA, Birns JW, et al. Laryngeal paralysis in children: a long-term retrospective study. Ann Otol Rhinol Laryngol 1982;91:417–24.
19. Kovesi T, Porcaro F, Petreschi F, et al. Vocal cord paralysis appears to be an acquired lesion in children with repaired esophageal atresia/tracheoesophageal fistula. Int J Pediatr Otorhinolaryngol 2018;112:45–7.
20. Lal DR, Gadepalli SK, Downard CD, et al. Challenging surgical dogma in the management of proximal esophageal atresia with distal tracheoesophageal fistula: outcomes from the Midwest Pediatric Surgery Consortium. J Pediatr Surg 2018;53:1267–72.
21. Hseu A, Recko T, Jennings R, et al. Upper airway anomalies in congenital tracheoesophageal fistula and esophageal atresia patients. Ann Otol Rhinol Laryngol 2015;124:808–13.
22. Demidchik YE, Demidchik EP, Reiners C, et al. Comprehensive clinical assessment of 740 cases of surgically treated thyroid cancer in children of Belarus. Ann Surg 2006;243:525–32.
23. Harness JK, Thompson NW, McLeod MK, et al. Differentiated thyroid carcinoma in children and adolescents. World J Surg 1992;16:547–53 [discussion: 553–4].
24. Scholz S, Smith JR, Chaignaud B, et al. Thyroid surgery at Children's Hospital Boston: a 35-year single-institution experience. J Pediatr Surg 2011;46:437–42.
25. Shrime M, Kacker A, Bent J, et al. Fourth branchial complex anomalies: a case series. Int J Pediatr Otorhinolaryngol 2003;67:1227–33.
26. Mandell DL. Head and neck anomalies related to the branchial apparatus. Otolaryngol Clin North Am 2000;33:1309–32.
27. Schumacher RE, Weinfeld IJ, Bartlett RH. Neonatal vocal cord paralysis following extracorporeal membrane oxygenation. Pediatrics 1989;84:793–6.
28. Neidich MJ, Prager JD, Clark SL, et al. Comprehensive airway management of neonatal head and neck teratomas. Otolaryngol Head Neck Surg 2011;144: 257–61.
29. Kikura M, Suzuki K, Itagaki T, et al. Age and comorbidity as risk factors for vocal cord paralysis associated with tracheal intubation. Br J Anaesth 2007;98:524–30.
30. Cavo JW Jr. True vocal cord paralysis following intubation. Laryngoscope 1985; 95:1352–9.
31. Jabbour J, North LM, Bougie D, et al. Vocal fold immobility due to birth trauma: a systematic review and pooled analysis. Otolaryngol Head Neck Surg 2017;157: 948–54.
32. de Gaudemar I, Roudaire M, Francois M, et al. Outcome of laryngeal paralysis in neonates: a long term retrospective study of 113 cases. Int J Pediatr Otorhinolaryngol 1996;34:101–10.

33. Emery PJ, Fearon B. Vocal cord palsy in pediatric practice: a review of 71 cases. Int J Pediatr Otorhinolaryngol 1984;8:147–54.
34. Polaner DM, Billet AL, Richardson MA. Cardiovocal syndrome. Pediatrics 1986; 78:380.
35. Robida A, Povhe B. Cardiovocal syndrome in an infant with a double outlet of the right ventricle. Eur J Pediatr 1988;148:15–6.
36. Zaki SA, Asif S, Shanbag P. Ortner syndrome in infants. Indian Pediatr 2010;47: 351–3.
37. Condon LM, Katkov H, Singh A, et al. Cardiovocal syndrome in infancy. Pediatrics 1985;76:22–5.
38. Rosin DF, Handler SD, Potsic WP, et al. Vocal cord paralysis in children. Laryngoscope 1990;100:1174–9.
39. Zur KB, Carroll LM. Recurrent laryngeal nerve reinnervation in children: acoustic and endoscopic characteristics pre-intervention and post-intervention. A comparison of treatment options. Laryngoscope 2015;125(Suppl 11):S1–15.
40. Friedman EM. Role of ultrasound in the assessment of vocal cord function in infants and children. Ann Otol Rhinol Laryngol 1997;106:199–209.
41. Ongkasuwan J, Ocampo E, Tran B. Laryngeal ultrasound and vocal fold movement in the pediatric cardiovascular intensive care unit. Laryngoscope 2017; 127:167–72.
42. Vats A, Worley GA, de Bruyn R, et al. Laryngeal ultrasound to assess vocal fold paralysis in children. J Laryngol Otol 2004;118:429–31.
43. Zapletal A, Kurland G, Boas SR, et al. Airway function tests and vocal cord paralysis in lung transplant recipients. Pediatr Pulmonol 1997;23:87–94.
44. Liu YC, Varier I, Ongkasuwan J. Use of audiometric measurement for assessment of vocal-fold function in postextubation infants. JAMA Otolaryngol Head Neck Surg 2017;143:908–11.
45. Grundfast KM, Harley E. Vocal cord paralysis. Otolaryngol Clin North Am 1989; 22:569–97.
46. Benjamin B. Technique of laryngoscopy. Int J Pediatr Otorhinolaryngol 1987;13: 299–313.
47. Wohl DL, Kilpatrick JK, Leshner RT, et al. Intraoperative pediatric laryngeal electromyography: experience and caveats with monopolar electrodes. Ann Otol Rhinol Laryngol 2001;110:524–31.
48. Koch BM, Milmoe G, Grundfast KM. Vocal cord paralysis in children studied by monopolar electromyography. Pediatr Neurol 1987;3:288–93.
49. Jacobs IN, Finkel RS. Laryngeal electromyography in the management of vocal cord mobility problems in children. Laryngoscope 2002;112:1243–8.
50. Scott AR, Chong PS, Randolph GW, et al. Intraoperative laryngeal electromyography in children with vocal fold immobility: a simplified technique. Int J Pediatr Otorhinolaryngol 2008;72:31–40.
51. Woo P, Arandia H. Intraoperative laryngeal electromyographic assessment of patients with immobile vocal fold. Ann Otol Rhinol Laryngol 1992;101:799–806.
52. Maturo SC, Braun N, Brown DJ, et al. Intraoperative laryngeal electromyography in children with vocal fold immobility: results of a multicenter longitudinal study. Arch Otolaryngol Head Neck Surg 2011;137:1251–7.
53. Engeseth MS, Olsen NR, Maeland S, et al. Left vocal cord paralysis after patent ductus arteriosus ligation: a systematic review. Paediatr Respir Rev 2018;27: 74–85.

54. Jabbour J, Martin T, Beste D, et al. Pediatric vocal fold immobility: natural history and the need for long-term follow-up. JAMA Otolaryngol Head Neck Surg 2014; 140:428–33.
55. Benjamin JR, Smith PB, Cotten CM, et al. Long-term morbidities associated with vocal cord paralysis after surgical closure of a patent ductus arteriosus in extremely low birth weight infants. J Perinatol 2010;30:408–13.
56. Tucker HM. Vocal cord paralysis in small children: principles in management. Ann Otol Rhinol Laryngol 1986;95:618–21.
57. Cantarella G, Viglione S, Forti S, et al. Voice therapy for laryngeal hemiplegia: the role of timing of initiation of therapy. J Rehabil Med 2010;42:442–6.
58. Schindler A, Bottero A, Capaccio P, et al. Vocal improvement after voice therapy in unilateral vocal fold paralysis. J Voice 2008;22:113–8.
59. Levine BA, Jacobs IN, Wetmore RF, et al. Vocal cord injection in children with unilateral vocal cord paralysis. Arch Otolaryngol Head Neck Surg 1995;121:116–9.
60. Cohen MS, Mehta DK, Maguire RC, et al. Injection medialization laryngoplasty in children. Arch Otolaryngol Head Neck Surg 2011;137:264–8.
61. Patel NJ, Kerschner JE, Merati AL. The use of injectable collagen in the management of pediatric vocal unilateral fold paralysis. Int J Pediatr Otorhinolaryngol 2003;67:1355–60.
62. Butskiy O, Mistry B, Chadha NK. Surgical interventions for pediatric unilateral vocal cord paralysis: a systematic review. JAMA Otolaryngol Head Neck Surg 2015;141:654–60.
63. Kimura M, Mau T, Chan RW. Viscoelastic properties of phonosurgical biomaterials at phonatory frequencies. Laryngoscope 2010;120:764–8.
64. Link DT, Rutter MJ, Liu JH, et al. Pediatric type I thyroplasty: an evolving procedure. Ann Otol Rhinol Laryngol 1999;108:1105–10.
65. Bouhabel S, Hartnick CJ. Current trends in practices in the treatment of pediatric unilateral vocal fold immobility: a survey on injections, thyroplasty and nerve reinnervation. Int J Pediatr Otorhinolaryngol 2018;109:115–8.
66. Smith ME, Roy N, Stoddard K. Ansa-RLN reinnervation for unilateral vocal fold paralysis in adolescents and young adults. Int J Pediatr Otorhinolaryngol 2008;72: 1311–6.
67. Paniello RC, Edgar JD, Kallogjeri D, et al. Medialization versus reinnervation for unilateral vocal fold paralysis: a multicenter randomized clinical trial. Laryngoscope 2011;121:2172–9.
68. Smith ME, Roy N, Houtz D. Laryngeal reinnervation for paralytic dysphonia in children younger than 10 years. Arch Otolaryngol Head Neck Surg 2012;138: 1161–6.
69. Smith ME, Houtz DR. Outcomes of laryngeal reinnervation for unilateral vocal fold paralysis in children: associations with age and time since injury. Ann Otol Rhinol Laryngol 2016;125:433–8.
70. Zur KB, Carroll LM. Recurrent laryngeal nerve reinnervation for management of aspiration in a subset of children. Int J Pediatr Otorhinolaryngol 2018;104:104–7.

Medications and Vocal Function

Jonathan M. Bock, MD

KEYWORDS

- Dysphonia • Medications • Anticholinergic • Reflux • Antipsychotic • Steroid inhaler

KEY POINTS

- Medications can induce changes in hydration state, direct laryngeal mucosal irritation, altered laryngeal muscle function, and induction of laryngeal hypersensitivity.
- Careful review of medication history and correlation of dysphonia symptoms with onset of medication therapy are necessary to detect deleterious medication effects on voice.
- Trials of medication reduction or avoidance can further clarify direct or indirect effects of medications on dysphonia symptoms.

The age of modern medicine in American is truly the age of polypharmacy. A majority of patients seen in the office of an otolaryngologist are prescribed numerous medications, and the rate of polypharmacy directly increases with the age of the patient.[1] Studies have shown the benefits in reducing the overall pharmaceutical burden to both the medical establishment at large and to the individual patient.[2] Patients often are prescribed inappropriate medications for hoarseness by primary care practitioners prior to visualization of the larynx, and rates of further medication utilization may be increased by otolaryngology providers on follow-up evaluation.[3,4] Medication side effects can be challenging to assess due to subtle timing of onset, additive effects of multiple medications in the same patient, and off-target or seemingly unrelated toxicity of treatments. Medication toxicity can happen from standard or even low-dose therapies with prescription or over-the-counter remedies. It, therefore, is crucial for the otolaryngologist to critically evaluate the medication regimen of the patient with dysphonia with particular attention to direct and indirect side-effect profiles of common medications.[5]

The range of potential side effects of medications on the larynx is broad but can be grouped into several specific categories:

Disclosure: Dr J.M. Bock is a paid consultant for Diversatek Healthcare, Milwaukee, WI, USA.
Division of Laryngology and Professional Voice, Department of Otolaryngology and Communication Sciences, Medical College of Wisconsin, 8701 Watertown Plank Road, Milwaukee, WI 53226, USA
E-mail address: jbock@mcw.edu

Otolaryngol Clin N Am 52 (2019) 693–702
https://doi.org/10.1016/j.otc.2019.03.013
0030-6665/19/© 2019 Elsevier Inc. All rights reserved.

oto.theclinics.com

Abbreviations	
ACE	Angiotensin-converting enzyme
ARB	Angiotensin receptor blocker
LPR	Laryngopharyngeal reflux
PPI	Proton pump inhibitor

- Antihistamines, diuretics, decongestants, antidepressants, and α-blockers used for benign prostatic hypertrophy all can contribute to laryngeal desiccation with concomitant vocal fatigue and dysphonia.
- Steroid inhalers and other inhaled medications can induce localized vocal fold inflammation and mucosal irritation as well as a predisposition for oropharyngeal and laryngeal infections.
- Antipsychotics, sedatives, and anticonvulsant medications can alter oropharyngeal and laryngeal muscle function, inducing laryngeal or esophageal tardive dyskinesia, dysarthria, or tremor.
- Hypertension medications, such as angiotensin-converting enzyme (ACE) inhibitors or angiotensin receptor blockers (ARBs), can induce laryngeal hypersensitivity and irritability syndromes manifested with throat clearing or chronic cough behaviors.

This article reviews currently available published data on risks of commonly used medication classes to induce changes in vocal function and suggests alternatives for treatment of patients with these unfortunate side effects.

STEROIDS

The short-term and long-term effects of steroids on patient mood, wound healing, and blood sugar levels are well known and likely already familiar to the otolaryngologist but are worthy of formal review because these medications are a regular adjunct for voice care. The risks of steroid use are additive over time in many cases and should be discussed with patients who may require repeated courses.[6] Recent reviews show that the most frequently rated complications of prolonged oral steroid use are incredibly common, with approximately half of all patients reporting some level of insomnia, mood disturbances, hyperphagia, and lipodystrophy. The rate of incidence of some adverse events (weight gain and easy bruising) seems to increase over time whereas some complications often occur quickly, such as insomnia or mood disorders.[7] Hyperglycemia can be severe after even small doses of oral steroids in some patients, due to the ability of steroids to inhibit adipocytes and hepatocytes to bind and process insulin.[8] Steroids inhibit neutrophil function through multiple mechanisms and can lead to higher rates of systemic infections and poor wound healing, especially in patients who are immunosuppressed. Corticosteroid-induced lipodystrophy with concomitant redistribution of adipose tissue (moon facies) also is common after prolonged oral steroid courses and can occur in up to 15% of patients after several months of treatment, even with doses as low as 10 mg per day of prednisone.[7] Bone loss also is common after prolonged steroid use but may be reversible once treatment is stopped.[9] Avascular necrosis of the hip is associated primarily with cumulative dose of steroids over time and is believed due to direct steroid inhibition of blood perfusion of the femoral neck. Rates may be as high as 0.3% after a mean dose of 673 mg of prednisone according to a recent review, which warrants consideration for any patients who may require larger or more prolonged dosing of oral steroids.[10] Steroids commonly induce posterior subcapsular cataract formation and can induce glaucoma in some patients, with subsequent visual field loss and optic nerve atrophy. It seems that cataract formation is again dependent on dose and duration of steroid administration.[11] Recent reviews have shown that intranasal steroids do not seem to have the same effect on cataract induction.[12] Corticosteroid administration was associated with increased rates of gastrointestinal ulceration and bleeding in a recent meta-analysis but only in hospitalized patients. Rates of ulceration leading to bleeding complications were uncommon in the ambulatory population and may increase with concomitant nonsteroidal anti-inflammatory drug dosing.[13] Adrenal suppression also may be of concern in some patients; however, clinically significant effects of corticosteroid dosing on the hypothalamic-pituitary-adrenal axis seem unlikely after short courses of oral steroids.[14] Psychiatric disturbances are highly variable after steroid treatment and can range from mild irritability to frank psychosis and mania. Recent reviews suggest that approximately 25% of patients experience mild mood changes on steroids, whereas severe complications are lower but still significant in approximately 5% of patients. Rates of psychiatric complications seem related primarily to dose, increasingly significantly at doses of more than 80 mg/d of prednisone. Studies have not been able to directly correlate prior psychiatric illness or mood disorders with increased rates of mood disorders after oral steroid administration.[15] These risks present a message of caution to the laryngologist to minimize dose and duration of oral steroid administration to minimize potential side effects.

Inhaled steroids often are used in the treatment of reactive airway disease and other inflammatory diseases of the lower respiratory tract and can induce direct contact effects on the tissues of the upper airway.[16] Oral and pharyngeal candidiasis are common issues for users of these preparations and may require ongoing treatment with antifungal preparations to prevent recurrence. High rates of dysphonia are reported after using nearly all inhaled steroid preparations, with dry powder formulations generally leading to higher rates of laryngeal irritation and inflammation. This is believed due directly to inhaled particle size, with higher rates of laryngeal deposition noted with larger inhaled particle sizes.[17] Fluticasone propionate (Advair) is particularly bothersome in this regard and laryngeal effects seem directly related to concentration and frequency of dosing.[18] Patients with advanced steroid inhaler laryngitis demonstrate bilateral midcord hyperkeratotic plaques with surrounding intense erythema and decreased mucosal wave propagation. Cessation of inhaled steroid preparations or change to other smaller-particle inhaled agents often are needed to resolve this localized inflammation (**Fig. 1**).[19] Ipratropium bromide, albuterol, and other inhaled

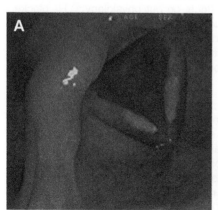 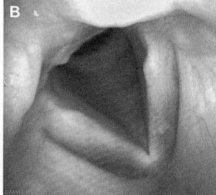

Fig. 1. (*A*) Severe steroid inhaler laryngitis. (*B*) Resolved steroid inhaler laryngitis following cessation of inhaled steroids for 3 months.

bronchodilators seem to have much less effect on vocal function but also may cause some localized inflammation at higher doses.[20]

REFLUX MEDICATIONS

Laryngopharyngeal reflux (LPR) has long been proposed as a cause of voice disorders, globus sensation, chronic cough, and mucus complaints in the otolaryngology patient population. Effects of reflux on voice are explored much more deeply in Dr Thomas L. Carroll's article, "Reflux and the Voice: Getting smarter about LPR," in this issue; this article focuses mainly on known side effects of reflux medications. Clinical research on LPR is challenging at best due to poor ability to screen for patients with pathologic proximal reflux issues using currently available technologies. Patient-based survey instruments, such as the reflux symptom index, seem to directly correlate with control of reflux symptoms with surgery and medication, whereas laryngeal examination–based surveys (such as the reflux finding score) do not seem to have significant reliability in clinical use.[21] Brief mention of side-effect profiles for commonly used medications for this issue is included for completeness.

Proton pump inhibitors (PPIs) are one of the most commonly prescribed medications in America and are commonly prescribed by primary care physicians for initial treatment of dysphonia.[22] Short courses of PPI are relatively safe, but studies have continued to present new risks of long-term PPI administration. Many of the risks of PPI use are believed to directly caused by the mechanism of PPIs, including hypomagnesemia, vitamin B_{12} deficiency, and small intestine bacterial overgrowth.[23] Risks of vitamin B_{12} deficiency have been seen to increase up to 65% in patients on long-term PPI treatment protocols, and rates of this increase with higher dose regimens.[24] Subsequent iron deficiency rates also have been shown to be elevated in patients on long-term PPI treatment protocols, suggesting that monitoring of anemia may also be appropriate in these patients.[25] There also have been many unclear disease associations published recently regarding chronic PPI use, including increased rates of bone fractures, Clostridium difficile infection, acute and chronic kidney disease, dementia, and community-acquired pneumonia.[23]

Histamine H_2-receptor antagonists (or H_2 blockers) have an even longer use history in otolaryngology than do PPIs and have some overlapping side-effect profiles, including risks of iron deficiency, bone metabolism alteration, vitamin B_{12} malabsorption, and increased rates of pneumonia. All of these are believed directly induced by alteration of gastric pH with downstream effects on gut physiology.[26] H_2 blockers also are known to cause a low rate of serious psychiatric side effects, such as mania and delirium, with higher rates in hospitalized patients and the elderly.[5] They remain a good option for patients who are not able to take PPIs due to potential interaction with coadministration of antiplatelet agents or documented PPI allergy.

ACETYLCHOLINESTERASE INHIBITORS

Associations with angiotension converting enzyme (ACE) inhibitors and cough are well established and have been acknowledged since these medications were first marketed and developed.[27] These medications are also known to have high risk of angioedema and unusual throat irritation symptoms that can develop at any time after initiation of therapy.[28] Only recently have large cohort studies shown that rates of cough may be much higher than previously reported in the pharmaceutical literature. Population-based studies have shown rates of cessation of ACE inhibitor therapy due to cough anywhere between 5% and 15%, and ARBs also can induce cough in this population.[29,30] It is, therefore, recommended that any patient with unusual throat irritation, fluctuating edema, dry cough, or other unexplained laryngeal symptoms has a trial of cessation of ACE or ARB therapy for several weeks to see if these symptoms resolve.

α_1-ADRENERGIC BLOCKERS

Rates of use of α_1-adrenergic blockers, such as tamsulosin, terazosin, doxazosin, and alfuzosin, for treatment of benign prostatic hypertrophy and overactive bladder have increased markedly over the past 20 years, and these medications are remarkably safe in clinical use. They also can be associated with significant xerostomia in many patients, and rates of this vary minimally between older and newer generations of these drugs. Dry mouth also is a main risk factor for patients on antimuscarinic therapies related to overactive bladder.[31] Xerostomia due to these agents can be severe and often is unable to be treated adequately with hydration or supplemental mouth rinses.[32]

PSYCHIATRIC MEDICATIONS

Psychiatric medication use has increased markedly over the past 20 years,[33] and these medications can be associated with multiple unwanted side effects, including weight gain, movement disorders, and xerostomia in up to 70% of patients.[34] Tricyclic antidepressants have been used for treatment of laryngeal sensory neuropathy for generations and can be associated with significant dry mouth complaints. Problematic xerostomia is an even more common side effect of many selective serotonin reuptake inhibitors and also been has described at markedly higher rates with serotonin-norepinephrine reuptake inhibitors.[35] These medications also increasingly are used for chronic pain and sensory neuropathy treatment protocols. Direct pooled meta-analysis data have shown lowest risk ratios for clinically significant xerostomia with citalopram use (a selective serotonin reuptake inhibitor), whereas venlafaxine and with serotonin-norepinephrine reuptake inhibitors in general have much higher rates of reported xerostomia.[35]

Antipsychotic medications are known to induce tardive dyskinesia and other related movement disorders in clinical practice and can have significant effects on laryngeal and esophageal motor function. These effects are seen less with atypical antipsychotic medications; they still can induce marked alterations in vocal cord movement and speech coordination.[36] Reports of bilateral vocal cord paralysis induction with stridor have been associated with risperidone treatment,[37] and speech precision and oropharyngeal ataxia can be induced by this medication as well.[38] Pooled meta-analysis data also have shown elevated rates of symptomatic dysphagia due to both typical and atypical antipsychotic medication administration.[39] It is fortunate these side effects of treatment often are reversible and can be improved by altered therapy regimens.[40] The otolaryngologist should rapidly communicate reported dysphonia and dysphagia complaints to a psychiatrist in these scenarios to facilitate improved quality of life for these patients.

ANTIHISTAMINES AND DECONGESTANTS

Most antihistamines and decongestants are purchased by patients over the counter and taken intermittently and, therefore, are difficult to monitor. They are commonly prescribed by primary care physicians for dysphonia due to possible allergic contributions to voice health.[4] These common household agents often have various medications combined in varying concentrations and it therefore can be challenging for a patient to fully realize the effects they may have on vocal quality. Preparations with pseudoephedrine are particularly responsible for xerostomia and should be avoided if possible for patients with laryngeal complaints.[41] Antihistamines as a class all induce sedation to varying degrees, with second-generation antihistamines more favorable in this regard.[42]

CAFFEINE

Caffeine has a storied history of avoidance among the laryngological intelligentsia due to potential risks of xerostomia, LPR, and subsequent dysphonia.[43] Data to support these associations are weak at best in the literature, and recent systematic reviews show no effects of caffeine on voice production.[44,45] Several well-done placebo-controlled clinical trials have shown no effect of moderate caffeine use on total body water or physiologic hydration state over several days of administration.[46,47] These data support the option for moderate use of caffeine in the vocal professional.

HORMONES

Testosterone-containing therapeutic androgen treatments often are used for treatment of endometriosis and postmenopausal sexual dysfunction and can induce significant vocal pitch lowering. This may be favorable for patients pursuing transgender transition but can be distressing if unwanted.[48] Studies show that transdermal preparations of low-dose testosterone have little effect on vocal pitch, but any complaint of vocal changes on these therapies should be taken seriously as voice changes may be irreversible.[49]

Estrogen replacement therapies seem to have much less risk for permanent voice change than testosterone-based supplemental therapies. Menstrual cycling is known to alter laryngeal vasculature and edema throughout the cycle, which may be altered by exogenous estrogens, and estrogen tone seems related to vocal quality later in life.[50] Estrogen-based hormone replacement therapies seem to preserve higher vocal range in women after menopause and may be a consideration for aging female vocal professional.[51]

PARKINSON DISEASE

Patients with Parkinson disease are known to have hypophonia due to vocal cord atrophy and poor vocal effort, along with peripheral tremor that interferes with gross motor movement. Patients with advanced multiple system atrophy also may progress to bilateral vocal cord immobility with progressive stridor.[52] Vocal cord augmentation with injectable agents may facilitate improved vocal closure for glottic atrophy associated with Parkinson disease,[53] but voice therapy remains the mainstay of long term vocal improvement for these patients.[54] Studies have shown that antiparkinsonism medications unfortunately have minimal effect on clinical vocal outcomes for patients with this disease.[55] Deep brain stimulation also seems to have minimal impact on vocal cord function for patients with advanced parkinsonism.[56]

HOMEOPATHIC MEDICATIONS

Use of homeopathic medications and dietary supplements continues at a high rate in the general population and among professional voice users.[57] Many common herbal supplements have known interaction with cytochrome P-450 processing of other medications, specifically St. John's wort. Ginkgo biloba is a known inducer of anticoagulation activity and should be avoided in singers and performers with concern for vocal hemorrhage. Ephedra can lead to arrhythmia at higher doses and also is implicated in dehydration and thickened laryngeal secretions.[58] Licorice products are proposed to have some antireflux effects but also can have hormonal activity and induce hypertension.[59] The voice care professional should carefully review all medications and supplements in their patients and discuss these possible side effects when appropriate.

REFERENCES

1. Salahudeen MS. Deprescribing medications in older people: a narrative review. Drugs of Today (Barc) 2018;54(8):489.
2. Maher RL, Hanlon J, Hajjar ER. Clinical consequences of polypharmacy in elderly. Expert Opin Drug Saf 2014;13(1):57–65.
3. Cohen SM, Lee H-J, Roy N, et al. Pharmacologic management of voice disorders by general medicine providers and otolaryngologists. Laryngoscope 2018; 128(3):682–9.
4. Cohen SM, Kim J, Roy N, et al. Prescribing patterns of primary care physicians and otolaryngologists in the management of laryngeal disorders. Otolaryngol Head Neck Surg 2013;149(1):118–25.
5. Abaza MM, Levy S, Hawkshaw MJ, et al. Effects of medications on the voice. Otolaryngol Clin North Am 2007;40(5):1081–90.
6. Poetker DM. Oral corticosteroids in the management of chronic rhinosinusitis with and without nasal polyps: risks and benefits. Am J Rhinol Allergy 2015;29(5): 339–42.
7. Morin C, Fardet L. Systemic glucocorticoid therapy: risk factors for reported adverse events and beliefs about the drug. A cross-sectional online survey of 820 patients. Clin Rheumatol 2015;34(12):2119–26.
8. Hirsch IB, Paauw DS. Diabetes management in special situations. Endocrinol Metab Clin North Am 1997;26(3):631–45. Avilable at: http://www.ncbi.nlm.nih.gov/pubmed/9314019. Accessed October 31, 2018.
9. van Staa TP, Leufkens HG, Cooper C, et al. The epidemiology of corticosteroid-induced osteoporosis: a meta-analysis. Osteoporos Int 2002;13(10):777–87.
10. Wong GKC, Poon WS, Chiu KH. Steroid-induced avascular necrosis of the HIP in neurosurgical patients: epidemiological study. ANZ J Surg 2005;75(6):409–10.
11. Carnahan MC, Goldstein DA. Ocular complications of topical, peri-ocular, and systemic corticosteroids. Curr Opin Ophthalmol 2000;11(6):478–83. Available at: http://www.ncbi.nlm.nih.gov/pubmed/11141645. Accessed October 31, 2018.
12. Valenzuela CV, Liu JC, Vila PM, et al. Intranasal corticosteroids do not lead to ocular changes: a systematic review and meta-analysis. Laryngoscope 2018. https://doi.org/10.1002/lary.27209.
13. Narum S, Westergren T, Klemp M. Corticosteroids and risk of gastrointestinal bleeding: a systematic review and meta-analysis. BMJ Open 2014;4(5):e004587.
14. LaRochelle GE, LaRochelle AG, Ratner RE, et al. Recovery of the hypothalamic-pituitary-adrenal (HPA) axis in patients with rheumatic diseases receiving low-dose prednisone. Am J Med 1993;95(3):258–64. Available at: http://www.ncbi.nlm.nih.gov/pubmed/8368224. Accessed October 31, 2018.
15. Kershner P, Wang-Cheng R. Psychiatric side effects of steroid therapy. Psychosomatics 1989;30(2):135–9.
16. DelGaudio JM. Steroid inhaler laryngitis: dysphonia caused by inhaled fluticasone therapy. Arch Otolaryngol Head Neck Surg 2002;128(6):677–81. Available at: http://www.ncbi.nlm.nih.gov/pubmed/12049563. Accessed October 3, 2018.

17. Perkins EL, Basu S, Garcia GJM, et al. Ideal particle sizes for inhaled steroids targeting vocal granulomas: preliminary study using computational fluid dynamics. Otolaryngol Head Neck Surg 2018;158(3):511–9.

18. Mirza N, Kasper Schwartz S, Antin-Ozerkis D. Laryngeal findings in users of combination corticosteroid and bronchodilator therapy. Laryngoscope 2004;114(9): 1566–9.

19. Leschke TM, Blumin JH, Bock JM. Diagnosis and laryngeal complications of Bordatella pertussis infection in the ambulatory adult population. Otolaryngol Head Neck Surg 2014;151(5). https://doi.org/10.1177/0194599814549316.

20. Erickson E, Sivasankar M. Evidence for adverse phonatory change following an inhaled combination treatment. J Speech Lang Hear Res 2010;53(1):75.

21. Cumpston EC, Blumin JH, Bock JM. Dual pH with multichannel intraluminal impedance testing in the evaluation of subjective laryngopharyngeal reflux symptoms. Otolaryngol Head Neck Surg 2016;155(6):1014–20.

22. Fisichella PM. Hoarseness and laryngopharyngeal reflux. JAMA 2015;313(18): 1853.

23. Nehra AK, Alexander JA, Loftus CG, et al. Proton pump inhibitors: review of emerging concerns. Mayo Clin Proc 2018;93(2):240–6.

24. Lam JR, Schneider JL, Zhao W, et al. Proton pump inhibitor and histamine 2 receptor antagonist use and vitamin B $_{12}$ deficiency. JAMA 2013;310(22):2435.

25. Lam JR, Schneider JL, Quesenberry CP, et al. Proton pump inhibitor and histamine-2 receptor antagonist use and iron deficiency. Gastroenterology 2017;152(4):821–9.e1.

26. Cook D, Guyatt G. Prophylaxis against upper gastrointestinal bleeding in hospitalized patients. N Engl J Med 2018;378(26):2506–16.

27. Dicpinigaitis PV. Angiotensin-converting enzyme inhibitor-induced cough. Chest 2006;129(1):169S–73S.

28. Humbert X, Alexandre J, Sassier M, et al. Long delay to onset of ACE inhibitors-induced cough: reason of difficult diagnosis in primary care? Eur J Intern Med 2017;37:e50–1.

29. Gokhale M, Girman C, Chen Y, et al. Comparison of diagnostic evaluations for cough among initiators of angiotensin converting enzyme inhibitors and angiotensin receptor blockers. Pharmacoepidemiol Drug Saf 2016;25(5):512–20.

30. de Oliveira JRJM, Otuki MF, Cabrini DA, et al. Involvement of the TRPV1 receptor in plasma extravasation in airways of rats treated with an angiotensin-converting enzyme inhibitor. Pulm Pharmacol Ther 2016;41:25–33.

31. Gacci M, Novara G, De Nunzio C, et al. Tolterodine extended release in the treatment of male oab/storage luts: a systematic review. BMC Urol 2014;14(1):84.

32. Tanasiewicz M, Hildebrandt T, Obersztyn I. Xerostomia of various etiologies: a review of the literature. Adv Clin Exp Med 2016;25(1):199–206.

33. Stagnitti MN. Trends in antidepressant utilization and expenditures in the U.S. civilian noninstitutionalized population by age, 2000 and 2010 2001. Available at: http://www.ncbi.nlm.nih.gov/pubmed/29360316. Accessed October 31, 2018.

34. Uher R, Farmer A, Henigsberg N, et al. Adverse reactions to antidepressants. Br J Psychiatry 2009;195(03):202–10.

35. Cappetta K, Beyer C, Johnson JA, et al. Meta-analysis: risk of dry mouth with second generation antidepressants. Prog Neuropsychopharmacol Biol Psychiatry 2018;84(Pt A):282–93.

36. Rowley H, Lynch T, Keogh I, et al. Tardive dystonia of the larynx in a quadriplegic patient: an unusual cause of stridor. J Laryngol Otol 2001;115(11):918–9.

Available at: http://www.ncbi.nlm.nih.gov/pubmed/11779311. Accessed October 3, 2018.

37. Ganesh M, Jabbar U, Iskander FH. Acute laryngeal dystonia with novel antipsychotics: a case report and review of literature. J Clin Psychopharmacol 2015; 35(5):613–5.

38. Sinha P, Vandana VP, Lewis NV, et al. Evaluating the effect of risperidone on speech: a cross-sectional study. Asian J Psychiatr 2015;15:51–5.

39. Miarons Font M, Rofes Salsench L. Antipsychotic medication and oropharyngeal dysphagia. Eur J Gastroenterol Hepatol 2017;29(12):1332–9.

40. Crouse EL, Alastanos JN, Bozymski KM, et al. Dysphagia with second-generation antipsychotics: a case report and review of the literature. Ment Health Clin 2017; 7(2):56–64.

41. Wellington K, Jarvis B. Cetirizine/pseudoephedrine. Drugs 2001;61(15):2231–40.

42. Ozdemir PG, Karadag AS, Selvi Y, et al. Assessment of the effects of antihistamine drugs on mood, sleep quality, sleepiness, and dream anxiety. Int J Psychiatry Clin Pract 2014;18(3):161–8.

43. Trinidade A, Robinson T, Phillips JS. The role of caffeine in otorhinolaryngology: guilty as charged? Eur Arch Otorhinolaryngol 2014;271(8):2097–102.

44. Franca MC, Simpson KO, Schuette A. Effects of caffeine on vocal acoustic and aerodynamic measures of adult females. Codas 2013;25(3):250–5. Available at: http://www.ncbi.nlm.nih.gov/pubmed/24408336. Accessed October 3, 2018.

45. Erickson-Levendoski E, Sivasankar M. Investigating the effects of caffeine on phonation. J Voice 2011;25(5):e215–9.

46. Silva AM, Júdice PB, Matias CN, et al. Total body water and its compartments are not affected by ingesting a moderate dose of caffeine in healthy young adult males. Appl Physiol Nutr Metab 2013;38(6):626–32.

47. Killer SC, Blannin AK, Jeukendrup AE. No evidence of dehydration with moderate daily coffee intake: a counterbalanced cross-over study in a free-living population. PLoS One 2014;9(1):e84154.

48. Baker J. A report on alterations to the speaking and singing voices of four women following hormonal therapy with virilizing agents. J Voice 1999;13(4):496–507. Available at: http://www.ncbi.nlm.nih.gov/pubmed/10622516. Accessed October 31, 2018.

49. Glaser R, York A, Dimitrakakis C. Effect of testosterone therapy on the female voice. Climacteric 2016;19(2):198–203.

50. Jost L, Fuchs M, Loeffler M, et al. Associations of sex hormones and anthropometry with the speaking voice profile in the adult general population. J Voice 2018; 32(3):261–72.

51. D'haeseleer E, Depypere H, Claeys S, et al. The impact of hormone therapy on vocal quality in postmenopausal women. J Voice 2012;26(5):671.e1-7.

52. Blumin JH, Berke GS. Bilateral vocal fold paresis and multiple system atrophy. Arch Otolaryngol Head Neck Surg 2002;128(12):1404–7. Available at: http://www.ncbi.nlm.nih.gov/pubmed/12479729. Accessed November 5, 2018.

53. Blumin JH, Pcolinsky DE, Atkins JP. Laryngeal findings in advanced Parkinson's disease. Ann Otol Rhinol Laryngol 2004;113(4):253–8.

54. Dashtipour K, Tafreshi A, Lee J, et al. Speech disorders in Parkinson's disease: pathophysiology, medical management and surgical approaches. Neurodegener Dis Manag 2018;8(5):337–48.

55. Cushnie-Sparrow D, Adams S, Abeyesekera A, et al. Voice quality severity and responsiveness to levodopa in Parkinson's disease. J Commun Disord 2018;76: 1–10.

56. Arocho-Quinones E, Hammer M, Bock J, et al. Effects of deep brain stimulation on vocal fold immobility in Parkinson's disease. Surg Neurol Int 2017;8(1):22.
57. Trivedi R, Salvo MC. Utilization and safety of common over-the-counter dietary/nutritional supplements, herbal agents, and homeopathic compounds for disease prevention. Med Clin North Am 2016;100(5):1089–99.
58. Lee JY, Jun SA, Hong SS, et al. Systematic review of adverse effects from herbal drugs reported in randomized controlled trials. Phytother Res 2016;30(9):1412–9.
59. Nazari S, Rameshrad M, Hosseinzadeh H. Toxicological effects of *Glycyrrhiza glabra* (licorice): a review. Phyther Res 2017;31(11):1635–50.

The White Lesion, Hyperkeratosis, and Dysplasia

S. Ahmed Ali, MD, Joshua D. Smith, BA, Norman D. Hogikyan, MD*

KEYWORDS

- Dysplasia • Larynx • Vocal fold • Leukoplakia • Erythroplakia • White lesion
- Laryngology

KEY POINTS

- Laryngeal mucosal precursor lesions often manifest as mucosal surface changes of leukoplakia, erythroplakia, or erythroleukoplakia, and may be symptomatic or asymptomatic.
- These gross mucosal changes may represent benign, premalignant, or malignant entities.
- Dysplastic lesions present a challenge because of the involved anatomic structures, risk of recurrence, or malignant progression.
- Multiple management options exist, with treatment decisions made jointly by physician and patient and focused on both appropriate lesion treatment and preservation of laryngeal structure and function.
- Research is ongoing to advance understanding of lesion biology and to optimize prevention and treatment.

BACKGROUND

A white lesion on a vocal fold is commonly encountered in the laryngology clinic and presents diagnostic and therapeutic challenges. Simply stated, clinicians are tasked with understanding the nature of the lesions as well as functional consequences associated with the disease or its treatment. These concepts may seem straightforward, but care is complicated by the fact that white lesions can represent asymptomatic, symptomatic, benign, premalignant, or malignant processes. The spectrum of laryngeal mucosal precursor lesions (LMPLs) spans the breadth of pathologic changes from hyperplasia or hyperkeratosis to severe dysplasia. This article focuses on vocal fold hyperkeratosis and dysplasia and explores the biology and clinical considerations associated with these and related conditions.

Disclosure: The authors have no financial interests to disclose.
Department of Otolaryngology – Head & Neck Surgery, Michigan Medicine, 1904 Taubman Center, 1500 East Medical Center Drive, Ann Arbor, MI 48109-5312, USA
* Corresponding author.
E-mail address: nhogikya@med.umich.edu

Otolaryngol Clin N Am 52 (2019) 703–712
https://doi.org/10.1016/j.otc.2019.03.014
oto.theclinics.com
0030-6665/19/© 2019 Elsevier Inc. All rights reserved.

GROSS CLASSIFICATION OF LARYNGEAL MUCOSAL PRECURSOR LESIONS

It is important to separate gross or macroscopic characterization of vocal fold lesions from histopathologic characterization because there is not a reliably predictable relationship. Macroscopic descriptors are used by clinicians to relay the gross appearance and can include leukoplakia (Greek, white patch), erythroplakia (Greek, red patch), and erythroleukoplakia.[1] Macroscopic alterations in vocal fold appearance are shown in **Fig. 1**. The incidence of dysplasia within leukoplakic lesions approximates 50%.[2] The rate of conversion to squamous cell carcinoma (SCC) is contingent on the extent and/or degree of dysplasia.[3] Clinical factors, such as absent mucosal wave, are also potentially predictive of shorter time to recurrence, although alteration of mucosal wave propagation is not reliably predictive of the presence of cancer.[4,5] A review on 1184 patients with vocal fold leukoplakia determined that within 6 months of initial diagnosis, 11% were diagnosed with laryngeal cancer.[6] Studies in the oral cavity literature describe an erythroplakia malignant transformation rate of 44.8%.[7]

HISTOLOGIC CLASSIFICATION OF LARYNGEAL MUCOSAL PRECURSOR LESIONS

Dysplasia is the histopathologic manifestation of mutation in normal epithelial cells and can include mitoses in higher layers of epithelium, nuclear structural abnormalities, and architectural changes.[8] Dysplasia grading remains an area of controversy and frequent update because of lack of intraobserver and interobserver reliability and reproducibility.[9,10] The 3 eminent classification systems are outlined in **Table 1** and include the World Health Organization (WHO) classification, squamous intraepithelial neoplasia (SIN) classification, and the Ljubljana classification (LC) of squamous intraepithelial lesions (SILs).

The WHO classification was developed in 2005 as a 4-point system, including squamous cell hyperplasia, mild dysplasia, moderate dysplasia, severe dysplasia, and carcinoma in situ.[11] Studies on observer variability of the WHO classification show unconvincing agreement rates (35.8% to 69%) and kappa values (0.15–0.70).[9,12–17] The SIN classification is also used; its primary distinguishing feature from the 4-point dysplasia system is that SIN 3 combines severe dysplasia and carcinoma in situ.[9] The LC was developed in 1977 to address classification of the epithelial hyperplastic laryngeal lesion.[18] Given ambiguity over the ideal system to use, pathologists attempted to

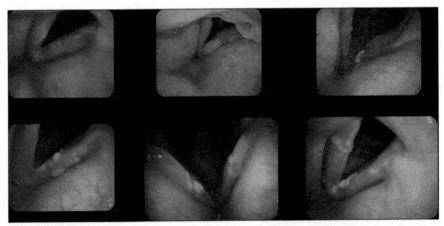

Fig. 1. Examples of laryngeal mucosal changes documented via videostroboscopy in clinic.

Table 1
Classification systems used for laryngeal mucosal precursor lesions

2005 WHO Classification	SIN	1971 Ljubljana Classification SIL	2016 Ljubljana Classification SIL	2017 WHO Classification
Squamous cell hyperplasia	—	Squamous hyperplasia	Low-grade dysplasia	Low-grade dysplasia
Mild dysplasia	SIN I	Basal/parabasal hyperplasia		
Moderate dysplasia	SIN II	Atypical hyperplasia	High-grade dysplasia	High-grade dysplasia
Severe dysplasia	SIN III			
Carcinoma in situ		Carcinoma in situ	Carcinoma in situ	Carcinoma in situ

Abbreviations: SIL, squamous intraepithelial lesion; SIN, squamous intraepithelial neoplasia; WHO, World Health Organization.

ascertain superiority of one of the 3 main systems; a study by Sarioglu and colleagues[19] showed no significant difference in inter-observer agreement for the WHO, LC, or SIN systems (0.42, 0.41, and 0.37 respectively). At the center of poor interobserver consistency was the category of moderate dysplasia.[16]

This lack of consistency drove reformation, because numerous studies advocated for a 2-tier grading system.[16,20] The LC was modified from significant differences in progression to malignancy rates between low-grade and high-grade groups, strengthening the prognostic value of the classification system.[21] This update prompted changes in the 2017 WHO guidelines, in which the scheme is low grade and high grade.[11,22] The update was accomplished via consolidation of moderate dysplasia, severe dysplasia, and carcinoma in situ into a high-grade dysplasia group.[22]

RISK FACTORS

The principal environmental causal factors implicated in driving development of LMPL, and subsequent laryngeal SCC, are tobacco use, alcohol abuse, and gastroesophageal reflux disease. Smoking has a greater causative effect than alcohol for laryngeal SCC, and carcinogenesis is related to direct irritation by the smoke.[23,24]

The risk conferred via gastroesophageal reflux is potentially unique to the larynx. Although the relationship has long been suspected, the associated risk has remained unclear because of poorly controlled studies.[25] Although recommending treatment of previously undiagnosed laryngopharyngeal reflux is beneficial from a nononcologic perspective, its possible chemoprevention role has not yet been fully elucidated.

GENETIC AND IMMUNOLOGIC BIOMARKERS OF LARYNGEAL MUCOSAL PRECURSOR LESIONS

Histopathologic assessment of dysplasia severity in LMPLs remains the standard for predicting risk of malignant transformation and need for timely treatment. However, traditional dysplasia grading systems are hindered by marked inter-rater and intrarater variability and suboptimal correlation between dysplasia severity and risk of malignancy.[20] Coupled with the importance of early detection of incident larynx SCC, this has prompted a search for predictive biomarkers of malignant progression in LMPLs; the results are summarized in **Table 2**.

Histologic progression from LMPL to invasive SCC is paralleled by accumulation of increasingly deleterious mutations in genes of the cell cycle (eg, CCND1, CDKN2A), apoptosis (eg, TP53), and growth signaling (eg, epidermal growth factor receptor

Table 2
Summary of genetic alterations shown to increase risk of laryngeal mucosal precursor lesion malignant transformation

Reference	Gene/ Chromosome	Gene Function	Alteration
Manterola et al,[26] 2018	FGFR3	Cell growth and proliferation	Point mutation, activating
	PIK3CA	Cell growth and proliferation	Point mutation, activating
	TP53	Apoptosis and cell-cycle regulation	Point mutation, inactivating
Bergshoeff et al,[27] 2014	Chromosome 1	—	Aneuploidy
	Chromosome 7	—	Aneuploidy
Liu et al,[28] 2012	TERC	Telomere maintenance	Gene amplification
Bartlett et al,[29] 2012	MMP-1, MMP-2, MMP-9	Extracellular matrix degradation and cell migration	Gene overexpression

[EGFR], phosphatidylinositol 4,5-bisphosphate 3-kinase catalytic subunit alpha [PIK3CA]) pathways (The Cancer Genome Atlas, 25631445). A recent case-control study found that mutations in the receptor tyrosine kinases FGFR3 and PIK3CA were present in LMPLs that progressed to invasive SCC but absent in nonprogressing lesions.[26] In contrast, mutations in the JAK3 and MET kinases and the ubiquitinating enzyme FBXW7 were exclusively found in nonprogressing LMPLs. The investigators concluded that these specific mutational profiles may be clinically useful biomarkers of malignant progression.

A few other genomic aberrations in LMPLs have been posited as potentially useful biomarkers for prognostication and treatment selection. Chromosomal instability, defined by aneuploidy of chromosomes 1 and 7, and amplification of the human telomerase RNA component (hTERC) gene are both robust predictors of LMPL malignant progression, even for lesions with mild dysplasia.[27,28] Similarly, overexpression of matrix metalloproteinases (MMP-1, MMP-2) responsible for extracellular matrix degradation and invasion seem to predict histologic progression of LMPLs.[29]

The view that specific genetic alterations may explain differential risk of malignant progression in LMPLs may only be a part of a larger, complex biological picture. Both genetic and immunologic biomarkers are likely to significantly improve the modest and inconsistent power of current histologic grading systems in predicting malignant progression of LMPLs. To realize this potential, large-scale genomic and immunologic studies of matched LMPLs and metachronous SCCs may be necessary.

DIAGNOSIS

Alterations in voice typically prompt in-office examination and identification of potential LMPLs of the vocal folds. The principles of diagnosis of vocal fold mucosal lesions involve a thorough history, vocal capabilities and voice-related quality of life assessments, head and neck examination, and laryngeal endoscopy.[30] Options for laryngeal examination include indirect mirror examination, flexible laryngoscopy, rigid endoscopy, and videostroboscopy.

Adjuncts to traditional laryngoscopy modalities may provide further insights into the nature of visualized lesions. A novel new technique combines flexible endoscopy with narrow-band imaging (NBI). NBI shows promise for differentiating benign from malignant lesions, with excellent specificity and sensitivity in detecting preneoplastic laryngeal lesions.[31,32] High-speed video of the larynx provides a more realistic visualization of vibratory movements of the vocal folds than stroboscopy, and holds promise for enhancing understanding of a lesion before tissue biopsy.[33,34] Endoscopic ultrasonography provides valuable adjunctive data regarding size and infiltration of laryngeal tumors.[35]

Once a potential LMPL is identified, further evaluation and tissue diagnosis are traditionally the next steps. The importance of tissue diagnosis is underscored by poor concordance between alterations in vibratory patterns detected on stroboscopy and presence of dysplasia.[36] With some lesions, initial tissue diagnosis may be combined with treatment through excisional biopsy. Microscopic direct laryngoscopy remains the gold standard for diagnosis. In-office biopsy is also possible for selected patients and lesions. Available methodologies for office-based procedures have evolved over time and are discussed later.

MANAGEMENT

Treatment armamentarium and philosophy evolve with time and vary by surgeon and institution, and some investigators have proposed structured guidelines for optimal management.[10,37,38] Discussion of management must acknowledge that laryngologists often simultaneously diagnose and treat white lesions in the larynx through excisional biopsy, and treatment may be designed to address multiple possible histologic subtypes; this is particularly true for lesions that are predicted to be on the lower end of the dysplasia spectrum. Diagnostic incisional biopsy as the sole goal of an initial procedure is also frequently performed and informs ensuing treatment. Furthermore, given the propensity for recurrent hyperkeratotic or dysplastic laryngeal lesions, management of subsequent lesions typically takes into consideration prior pathology reports while also recognizing that lesion evolution can occur. A variety of treatment modalities available to contemporary laryngologists is discussed here.

Conservative and Medical Management

Expectant observation with conservative medical management may be considered for select patients. For patients who are immunosuppressed from an innate or iatrogenic perspective, particularly those on potent inhaled steroids, the possibility of candidiasis should be considered for lesions that are not clearly neoplastic.[39]

Asymptomatic or minimally symptomatic lesions, particularly in vocal professionals, for which significant dysphonia is anticipated postexcision may in some cases be observed following discussion of options and if the patient will reliably return for follow-up. In all cases in which conservative management is used, close follow-up is crucial and the threshold for definitive treatment must remain low.

Microsurgical Excision

Use of surgical treatment of dysplasia is heavily practitioner dependent. However, surgical excision is the historical standard by which other treatment methods are judged. Both laser and cold-steel excision techniques are used, with CO_2 laser being the traditional workhorse laser in the larynx. The benefits of using CO_2 laser include superior hemostatic capabilities, better anatomic preservation, and enhanced precision of action.[40] Although there have been concerns regarding thermal burns potentially affecting surgical margin analysis and deeper surgical wounds with CO_2 excision, differences in wound healing have not been shown in case-controlled studies.[41] The potassium titanyl phosphate (KTP) laser is being increasingly used in the operating room;

early studies have shown equivalent results to CO_2 excision and potential superiority to the pulsed dye laser (PDL).[42,43] Additional details regarding the 532-nm laser are presented later.

Recurrence rates for low-grade to moderate-grade dysplasia treated via either cold-steel endoscopic excision or CO_2 laser excision range from 8% to 29%.[44–47] Extent of malignant progression following management of low-grade to moderate-grade dysplasia with surgical excision ranges from 0% to 35%.[44,46,48] The specific surgical procedure to perform depends on degree of dysplasia, extent of dysplasia, and practitioner preference. When performing surgical excision, studies have shown that histologic examination confirmed frozen section in 95% of interventions for laryngeal tumors (including dysplasia).[49]

In-office Surgical Techniques

The introduction of working channel laryngoscopes paired with flexible waveguide–enabled lasers instruments has expanded the scope of in-office surgical techniques for diagnostic or therapeutic purposes. Proponents of this paradigm tout its reliability, safety, time-effectiveness, and cost-effectiveness, as well as reduced time to treatment.[50–53] There is controversy regarding utility of in-office biopsies of premalignant or malignant lesions because studies have shown a sensitivity of 60% for those categories.

Photoangiolytic lasers permit potential complete excision or ablation of LMPLs while preserving the underlying lamina propria, thus affording potential cure while maintaining vocal fold pliability and glottic closure.[54] The KTP laser is in widespread use, and use of this, PDL, or the CO_2 laser for ablative treatment of LMPLs is reported.[42] This technique affords potentially high rates of durable disease regression and cure with stability or improvement in voice.[55,56] However, ablative surgery for LMPLs necessitates surgical expertise, trained personnel, and maintenance of costly technology. Shortcomings include inability to examine pathologic specimens in procedures in which ablation only is performed, as well as potential for incomplete or inadequate treatment compared with operative surgical techniques.[10,42,45] It remains to be seen whether the newer lasers will widely supplant more proven laser systems. Further comparison studies are needed to determine optimum surgical tools and techniques.

Radiation

Radiotherapy (RT) remains a highly effective treatment option for early (ie, stage I and II) glottic cancers.[57] However, its use in treatment of LMPLs is limited, although some investigators advocate definitive RT for LMPLs in patients with multiply recurrent or extensive disease, those who continue to use tobacco, or those with high-risk comorbidities precluding anesthesia.[38]

Other Treatments

Photodynamic therapy is used for oral or laryngeal dysplasia. It has shown promising results as a treatment alternative for laryngeal dysplasia and early carcinoma with few permanent effects, although randomized clinical trial data are lacking and temporary photosensitivity is a significant shortcoming.[58,59]

Chemoprevention for dysplastic lesions is exciting because of its potential for treating dysplastic lesions and any existing field cancerization effect. Although numerous studies have shown promising preliminary results with folate supplementation, administration of bioactive agents such as interferon-alfa, alpha-tocopherol, and/or administration of retinoids, these agents do carry systemic effects.[60] Further research will continue to determine the role of biochemopreventive protocols in managing LMPLs.

SUMMARY

LMPLs may present because of an alteration in laryngeal function, most typically dysphonia, or be discovered as an asymptomatic but visible mucosal lesion. Overlying mucosal changes can manifest as leukoplakia, erythroplakia, or erythroleukoplakia; the spectrum of histopathologic changes present within any of these can involve simple hyperkeratosis to invasive carcinoma. Management options are practitioner and patient dependent, and informed by degree and extent of pathologic changes, symptoms, patient comorbidities, and their functional goals. Treatment tools include traditional measures such as surgical excision either via cold instruments or CO_2 laser. Newer options include photoablation via angiolytic lasers such as pulsed KTP or PDL. Novel therapies are being studied, including potential biochemopreventive substances. Given a propensity for recurrence or malignant progression despite the current treatment armamentarium, there remains room for improvement and innovation in the prevention, diagnosis, and management of the laryngeal white lesion.

REFERENCES

1. Ferlito A, Devaney KO, Woolgar JA, et al. Squamous epithelial changes of the larynx: diagnosis and therapy. Head Neck 2012;34(12):1810–6.
2. Isenberg JS, Crozier DL, Dailey SH. Institutional and comprehensive review of laryngeal leukoplakia. Ann Otol Rhinol Laryngol 2008;117(1):74–9.
3. Lee DH, Yoon TM, Lee JK, et al. Predictive factors of recurrence and malignant transformation in vocal cord leukoplakia. Eur Arch Otorhinolaryngol 2015; 272(7):1719–24.
4. Cui W, Xu W, Yang Q, et al. Clinicopathological parameters associated with histological background and recurrence after surgical intervention of vocal cord leukoplakia. Medicine (Baltimore) 2017;96(22):e7033.
5. Colden D, Jarboe J, Zeitels SM, et al. Stroboscopic assessment of vocal fold keratosis and glottic cancer. Ann Otol Rhinol Laryngol 2001;110(4):293–8.
6. Kostev K, Jacob L, Kalder M, et al. Association of laryngeal cancer with vocal cord leukoplakia and associated risk factors in 1,184 patients diagnosed in otorhinolaryngology practices in Germany. Mol Clin Oncol 2018;8(5):689–93.
7. Villa A, Villa C, Abati S. Oral cancer and oral erythroplakia: an update and implication for clinicians. Aust Dent J 2011;56(3):253–6.
8. Van Hulst AM, Kroon W, Van Der Linden ES, et al. Grade of dysplasia and malignant transformation in adults with premalignant laryngeal lesions. Head Neck 2016;38:E2284–90.
9. Fleskens S, Slootweg P. Grading systems in head and neck dysplasia: their prognostic value, weaknesses and utility. Head Neck Oncol 2009;1:11.
10. Mehanna H, Paleri V, Robson A, et al. Consensus statement by otorhinolaryngologists and pathologists on the diagnosis and management of laryngeal dysplasia. Clin Otolaryngol 2010;35(3):170–6.
11. Gale N, Poljak M, Zidar N. Update from the 4th edition of the World Health Organization classification of head and neck tumours: what is new in the 2017 WHO blue book for tumours of the hypopharynx, larynx, trachea and parapharyngeal space. Head Neck Pathol 2017;11(1):23–32.

12. Fischer DJ, Epstein JB, Morton TH Jr, et al. Interobserver reliability in the histopathologic diagnosis of oral pre-malignant and malignant lesions. J Oral Pathol Med 2004;33(2):65–70.

13. Tabor MP, Braakhuis BJM, van der Wal JE, et al. Comparative molecular and histological grading of epithelial dysplasia of the oral cavity and the oropharynx. J Pathol 2003;199(3):354–60.

14. Abbey LM, Kaugars GE, Gunsolley JC, et al. Intraexaminer and interexaminer reliability in the diagnosis of oral epithelial dysplasia. Oral Surg Oral Med Oral Pathol Oral Radiol 1995;80(2):188–91.

15. Karabulut A, Reibel J, Therkildsen MH, et al. Observer variability in the histologic assessment of oral premalignant lesions. J Oral Pathol Med 1995;24(5):198–200.

16. McLaren KM, Burnett RA, Goodlad JR, et al. Consistency of histopathological reporting of laryngeal dysplasia. Histopathology 2000;37(5):460–3.

17. Kujan O, Khattab A, Oliver RJ, et al. Why oral histopathology suffers interobserver variability on grading oral epithelial dysplasia: an attempt to understand the sources of variation. Oral Oncol 2007;43(3):224–31.

18. Gale N, Kambic V, Michaels L, et al. The Ljubljana classification: a practical strategy for the diagnosis of laryngeal precancerous lesions. Adv Anat Pathol 2000; 7(4):240–51.

19. Sarioglu S, Cakalagaoglu F, Elagoz S, et al. Inter-observer agreement in laryngeal pre-neoplastic lesions. Head Neck Pathol 2010;4(4):276–80.

20. Gale N, Blagus R, El-Mofty SK, et al. Evaluation of a new grading system for laryngeal squamous intraepithelial lesions-a proposed unified classification. Histopathology 2014;65(4):456–64.

21. Gale N, Gnepp DR, Poljak M, et al. Laryngeal squamous intraepithelial lesions: an updated review on etiology, classification, molecular changes, and treatment. Adv Anat Pathol 2016;23(2):84–91.

22. Cho KJ, Song JS. Recent changes of classification for squamous intraepithelial lesions of the head and neck. Arch Pathol Lab Med 2018;142(7):829–32.

23. Elwood JM, Pearson JCG, Skippen DH, et al. Alcohol, smoking, social and occupational factors in the aetiology of cancer of the oral cavity, pharynx and larynx. Int J Cancer 1984;34(5):603–12.

24. Brugere J, Guenel P, Leclerc A, et al. Differential effects of tobacco and alcohol in cancer of the larynx, pharynx, and mouth. Cancer 1986;57(2):391–5.

25. Qadeer MA, Colabianchi N, Strome M, et al. Gastroesophageal reflux and laryngeal cancer: causation or association? A critical review. Am J Otolaryngol 2006; 27(2):119–28.

26. Manterola L, Aguirre P, Larrea E, et al. Mutational profiling can identify laryngeal dysplasia at risk of progression to invasive carcinoma. Sci Rep 2018;8(1):6613.

27. Bergshoeff VE, Van Der Heijden SJA, Haesevoets A, et al. Chromosome instability predicts progression of premalignant lesions of the larynx. Pathology 2014;46(3):216–24.

28. Liu Y, Dong XL, Tian C, et al. Human telomerase RNA component (hTERC) gene amplification detected by FISH in precancerous lesions and carcinoma of the larynx. Diagn Pathol 2012;7(1):34.

29. Bartlett RS, Heckman WW, Isenberg J, et al. Genetic characterization of vocal fold lesions: leukoplakia and carcinoma. Laryngoscope 2012;122(2):336–42.

30. Hogikyan ND, Sethuraman G. Validation of an instrument to measure voice-related quality of life (V-RQOL). J Voice 1999;13(4):557–69.

31. Yang Y, Fang J, Zhong Q, et al. The value of narrow band imaging combined with stroboscopy for the detection of applanate indiscernible early-stage vocal cord cancer. Acta Otolaryngol 2018;138(4):400–6.

32. Watanabe A, Taniguchi M, Tsujie H, et al. The value of narrow band imaging for early detection of laryngeal cancer. Eur Arch Otorhinolaryngol 2009;266(7): 1017–23.

33. Popolo PS. Investigation of flexible high-speed video nasolaryngoscopy. J Voice 2018;32(5):529–37.

34. Hertegård S, Larsson H. A portable high-speed camera system for vocal fold examinations. J Voice 2014;28(6):681–7.

35. Arens C, Malzahn K, Dias O, et al. Endoscopic imaging techniques in the diagnosis of laryngeal cancer and its precursor lesions. Laryngorhinootologie 1999; 78(12):685–91.

36. Djukic V, Milovanovic J, Jotic AD, et al. Stroboscopy in detection of laryngeal dysplasia effectiveness and limitations. J Voice 2014;28(2):262.e13–21.

37. Karatayli-Ozgursoy S, Pacheco-Lopez P, Hillel AT, et al. Laryngeal dysplasia, demographics, and treatment: a single-institution, 20-year review. JAMA Otolaryngol Head Neck Surg 2015;141(4):313–8.

38. Cosway B, Paleri V. Laryngeal dysplasia: an evidence-based flowchart to guide management and follow up. J Laryngol Otol 2015;129(6):598–9.

39. Pabuççuoğlu U, Tuncer C, Sengiz Ş. Histopathology of candidal hyperplastic lesions of the larynx. Pathol Res Pract 2002;198(10):675–8.

40. Chen M, Chen J, Cheng L, et al. Recurrence of vocal fold leukoplakia after carbon dioxide laser therapy. Eur Arch Otorhinolaryngol 2017;274(9):3429–35.

41. Zhang Y, Liang G, Sun N, et al. Comparison of CO_2laser and conventional laryngomicrosurgery treatments of polyp and leukoplakia of the vocal fold. Int J Clin Exp Med 2015;8(10):18265–74.

42. Xie X, Young J, Kost K, et al. KTP 532 nm laser for laryngeal lesions. A systematic review. J Voice 2013;27(2):245–9.

43. Zeitels SM, Akst LM, Burns JA, et al. Office-based 532-nm pulsed KTP laser treatment of glottal papillomatosis and dysplasia. Ann Otol Rhinol Laryngol 2006; 115(9 I):679–85.

44. Leirens J, Vidts G, Schmelzer B, et al. Premalignant lesions of the vocal cords: a retrospective study of 62 cases treated with CO_2laser. Acta Otolaryngol 1997; 117(6):903–8.

45. Panwar A, Lindau R, Wieland A. Management of premalignant lesions of the larynx. Expert Rev Anticancer Ther 2013;13(9):1045–51.

46. Dispenza F, De Stefano A, Marchese D, et al. Management of laryngeal precancerous lesions. Auris Nasus Larynx 2012;39(3):280–3.

47. Mannelli G, Cecconi L, Gallo O. Laryngeal preneoplastic lesions and cancer: challenging diagnosis. Qualitative literature review and meta-analysis. Crit Rev Oncol Hematol 2016;106:64–90.

48. Ahn A, Wang L, Slaughter JC, et al. Serial full-thickness excision of dysplastic vocal fold leukoplakia: diagnostic or therapeutic? Laryngoscope 2015;126(4): 923–7.

49. Remacle M, Matar N, Delos M, et al. Is frozen section reliable in transoral CO2 laser-assisted cordectomies? Eur Arch Otorhinolaryngol 2010;267(3):397–400.

50. Lippert D, Hoffman MR, Dang P, et al. In-office biopsy of upper airway lesions: safety, tolerance, and effect on time to treatment. Laryngoscope 2015;125(4): 919–23.

51. Wellenstein DJ, Schutte HW, Takes RP, et al. Office-based procedures for the diagnosis and treatment of laryngeal pathology. J Voice 2018;32(4):502–13.
52. Cohen JT, Safadi A, Fliss DM, et al. Reliability of a transnasal flexible fiberoptic in-office laryngeal biopsy. JAMA Otolaryngol Head Neck Surg 2013;139(4):341–5.
53. Rosen CA, Amin MR, Sulica L, et al. Advances in office-based diagnosis and treatment in laryngology. Laryngoscope 2009;119(SUPPL. 2):S185–212.
54. Kishimoto Y, Suzuki R, Kawai Y, et al. Photocoagulation therapy for laryngeal dysplasia using angiolytic lasers. Eur Arch Otorhinolaryngol 2016;273(5):1221–5.
55. Koss SL, Baxter P, Panossian H, et al. Serial in-office laser treatment of vocal fold leukoplakia: disease control and voice outcomes. Laryngoscope 2017;127(7): 1644–51.
56. Fink DS, Sibley H, Kunduk M, et al. Subjective and objective voice outcomes after transoral laser microsurgery for early glottic cancer. Laryngoscope 2016;126(2): 405–7.
57. Stokes WA, Abbott D, Phan A, et al. Patterns of care for patients with early-stage glottic cancer undergoing definitive radiation therapy: a national cancer database analysis. Int J Radiat Oncol Biol Phys 2017;98(5):1014–21.
58. Rigual NR, Thankappan K, Cooper M, et al. Photodynamic therapy for head and neck dysplasia and cancer. Arch Otolaryngol Head Neck Surg 2009;135(8): 784–8.
59. Sadri M, McMahon J, Parker A. Management of laryngeal dysplasia: a review. Eur Arch Otorhinolaryngol 2006;263(9):843–52.
60. Mesolella M, Iengo M, Testa D, et al. Chemoprevention using folic acid for dysplastic lesions of the larynx. Mol Clin Oncol 2017;7(5):843–6.

Transgender Voice and Communication

Mingyang L. Gray, MD, MPH*, Mark S. Courey, MD

KEYWORDS

• Transgender • Voice • Phonosurgery • Fundamental frequency

KEY POINTS

- Hormone therapy has a greater effect on voice for female-to-male patients than male-to-female patients and should be in use for at least 6 months before considering significant intervention for voice and communication.
- Behavioral changes in style of communication and voice are the first-line treatment of transgender patients who wish to better match their perceived voice to their gender identity.
- Voice therapy should be offered to all transgender patients who demonstrate inefficient voice use.
- Phonosurgery is often a necessary adjunct to help patients reach their optimal voice.
- Female-to-male patients are underrepresented in the voice literature and likely are an undertreated population.

INTRODUCTION

The exact prevalence of transgender people is unknown but is estimated to be between 0% to 5% and 1% to 3% among birth-assigned (cis) men and between 0% to 4% and 1% to 2% among birth-assigned (cis) women.[1] Transgender patients often work with a multidisciplinary team to alter various aspects of their physical appearance and function to match their gender identity. There are many aspects of gender reassignment, including hormone therapy, psychosocial support, sexual reassignment surgery, voice therapy, and voice surgery.

For most people, voice allows for immediate identification of one's gender, age, and background. One objective difference between male and female voice that is easily measured is fundamental frequency (vocal pitch). The relative ease with which objective measures of pitch can be recorded has led many patients, clinicians, and

Disclosure Statement: The authors have no funding, financial relationships, or conflicts of interest to disclose.
Department of Otolaryngology–Head and Neck Surgery, Icahn School of Medicine at Mount Sinai, One Gustave L Levy Place – Box 1189, New York, NY 10029, USA
* Corresponding author.
E-mail address: mingyang.gray@mountsinai.org

Otolaryngol Clin N Am 52 (2019) 713–722
https://doi.org/10.1016/j.otc.2019.03.007   oto.theclinics.com
0030-6665/19/Published by Elsevier Inc.

researchers to focus on pitch as the main or sole outcome measure in patients during gender transition. Studies have reported stereotypical ranges in pitch among male speakers (between 100 and 120 Hz) and female speakers (between 190 and 220 Hz).[2] A gender-ambiguous pitch range has also been defined as F0 between 145 and 165 Hz.[3,4] Therefore, during transition, many patients and clinicians focus on obtaining pitch within gender-ambiguous ranges and male-to-female (MtF) patients aim for F0 greater than 150 to 160 Hz, whereas female-to-male (FtM) patients aim for F0 less than 150 Hz.

Traditionally, the approach of transgender patients and the clinicians who treat them has been on shifting the patients' fundamental frequency (F0), or the pitch of their voice. However, gender identification of voice relies on many other verbal and nonverbal behaviors.[5] Because of the complex multifaceted nature of voice and communication, having a higher or lower F0 alone does not always produce a voice congruent with the desired gender.[6] As such, successful behavioral therapy to help transition the "voice" in transgender patients must also address other aspects of communication, such as airflow, resonance or formant ranges, intonation, and intensity, as well as nonverbal communication and cultural norms (pragmatics). In general, voices perceived as feminine exhibit greater pitch range variability, lower intensity (loudness), and breathy quality. In contrast, voices perceived as masculine are more monotone with less range in pitch and greater intensity.[7,8] In a study that analyzed the intonation of cisgender and transgender patients, there were no significantly different intonation patterns. Intonation shift was defined as a change in 2 semitones, which are converted from frequency measured in Hertz. However, a higher frequency of upward intonation is perceived as a female behavior and can be used by transgender patients to influence gender perception.[6,9] Another study found that MtF patients who were identified as women had higher speaking formant frequencies (FF) and higher upper limit of speaking fundamental frequency.[6] Voice therapy builds the foundation for efficiently transitioning voice such that patients can live and be perceived as their gender identity.

Patient satisfaction with voice results and patient-reported outcomes are important measurements of success for transgender patients. Many different methods of measuring subjective results have been used by different researchers. Until recently, however, patient-reported outcomes measures were not specific for transgender voice and communication. The Transsexual Voice Questionnaire (TVQ^MtF) was validated as a patient-reported outcomes measurement tool with 3 categories: anxiety and avoidance, gender identity, and voice quality.[10,11] A lower total score represents a more desirable outcome. However, the TVQ^MtF has only been validated for MtF patients. Validation was accomplished by demonstrating internal consistency and reliability when compared with Transgender Self-evaluation Questionnaire (TSEQ). The TSEQ was developed based on the validated Voice Handicap Index. The TVQ^MtF has been further demonstrated to have internal consistency in a recent validity and reliability study.[11] Although an FtM corollary to the TVQ has been used in the literature, there are no current studies that have demonstrated validity for the TVQ^FtM.[12] The psychosocial stress associated with gender dysphoria, albeit outside the scope of this discussion, can also affect the quality of the transgender voice and should not be overlooked.[7,8] Future studies will be able to measure standardized subjective outcomes throughout the transitioning process.

MALE-TO-FEMALE TRANSITION

Most patients seen in the laryngology practice are MtF patients, which is comparable to their representation in medical literature.[8,13] Male puberty results in changes in the pharyngeal size, the laryngeal framework, and vocal fold development as a response to testosterone exposure. At a minimum, testosterone stimulates growth of the pharynx, the laryngeal framework, and thickening or increase in mass of the vocal folds, which results in lowering of FF and vocal pitch. Once the testosterone is withdrawn, however, muscle and mucosal atrophy is only minimal, and the formant ranges and vocal pitch are not significantly altered. MtF patients must develop methods to compensate for these changes. Again, because absolute pitch is easy to measure, patients and clinicians have traditionally focused on elevation of pitch during vocal modification. Pitch elevation, however, may sometimes harm the overall vocal production mechanism.[14] As a result of attempting to elevate pitch, MtF patients may be susceptible to voice disorders related to inefficient muscle tension patterns and may need more intervention to be fully perceived as a woman. Individual patient goals, such as living part time or full time as a woman, may influence intervention plans.

Hormone Therapy

For MtF transgender patients, hormone therapy rarely leads to the development of significant female voice characteristics because of irreversible structural changes to the larynx that have already occurred during male puberty.[3,12] In a study that followed the self-perception of voice as indicated by TVQ scores of transgender patients during the first year of hormone therapy, there was no association between hormone level and voice quality among MtF patients. Although all transgender patients reported an improvement in their voice, based on TVQ scores, after a year of hormone therapy, the underlying reason for these improvements for MtF patients was unclear. Unlike FtM patients, there was no linear correlation between serum testosterone levels and TVQ scores. Self-perception of voice may also be influenced by other effects of hormone therapy, such as breast development and living as a woman.[12] Because of these changes, it is recommended that patients receive hormone therapy for at least 6 months before further voice intervention. Many MtF patients require initial or sustained voice therapy with or without phonosurgery to achieve a satisfactory voice.

Voice Therapy

There are many variations of techniques and strategies to obtain and maintain a feminine voice. These variations are in part due to the complex nature of an individual's baseline and voice goals as well as a lack of standardized treatment among speech pathologists. One retrospective review of 25 MtF patients described a range of voice therapy programs tailored to the needs of individual patients.[2] Specific goals of voice therapy address issues such as phonotrauma, voice hygiene, pitch, intonation, resonance, and nonverbal communication. Techniques used include behavior therapy, such as flow phonation, to produce an efficient voice production on exhalation and resonant voice therapy to promote a target sound vibration through the oral cavity. Carew and colleagues[15] described voice therapy that focused on lip spreading and forward tongue carriage to feminize oral resonance. Many clinicians recommend that voice therapy start with practicing targeted frequency production and stabilized voice quality and move on to target phrases, sentences, and ultimately, culminate with multisentence communication.

The inefficient use of voice among MtF patients has been measured objectively. In an aerodynamic analysis of MtF voice production, the production of a female voice by MtF patients was associated with a higher maximum flow declination rate,[14] which is frequently seen in patients with hyperadduction voice disorders. Furthermore, the study confirmed that MtF patients exhibit incomplete closure of vocal folds to achieve a breathy voice. This altered closure pattern is often obtained through active separation of the vocal folds, which requires inefficient muscle use patterns rather than the more physiologic process of confidential voice use.

Efficient voice use with improved intonation, resonance, and behavior changes can change the way one's voice is perceived. One study showed that despite achieving a female pitch after undergoing Wendler glottoplasty (a surgical procedure that increases pitch by shortening the vocal folds; **Fig. 1**), some MtF patients continue to be misperceived on the telephone.[16] This study highlights the importance of voice beyond pitch. Resonance, as measured by FF, has also been proposed to shift the perception of gender. FFs are determined by the length, shape, and the size of the proximal and distal openings of the pharynx and oral cavity. The space within the pharynx and oral cavity can be made larger or smaller by moving the tongue anteriorly or posteriorly. In general, MtF patients with voice that is perceived to be a female voice tend to have higher FFs.[6] In 1 study, 10 MtF patients participated in 5 weekly therapy sessions targeting oral resonance techniques. Participants were able to achieve

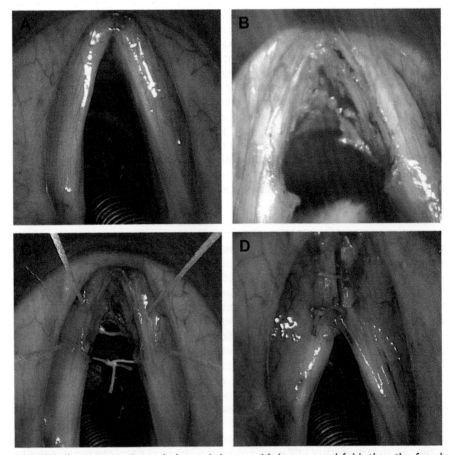

Fig. 1. (*A*) The preoperative male larynx is larger with longer vocal folds than the female larynx. (*B*) The anterior third of the vocal fold is deepithelialized. (*C*) Sutures are passed across both true vocal folds. (*D*) Absorbable sutures are secured to approximate the anterior third of the true vocal folds using endoscopic technique. (*Courtesy of* M. S. Courey, MD, New York, NY.)

increases in all FFs. There was improvement in listener ratings and self-perception of vocal femininity.[15] Another study reported manipulating computerized voice samples to increase the FFs of each vowel without increasing F0. Listeners perceived the samples with manipulated FFs as more feminine.[17]

The current literature demonstrates that voice therapy successfully results in vocal feminization with and without phonosurgery. However, 1-year follow-up reveals that early gains in terms of feminization and pitch elevation are not sustained, and longer-term outcomes are still lacking. There is one longitudinal study that followed 5 MtF patients for 15 months. Immediately after 8 weeks of voice therapy, perception of female gender improved approximately 50% of the time. After 15 months, the perception of female gender decreased to 33% of the time.[4] Despite all patients being perceived as more feminine, there was a wide range of responses to voice therapy. A study that compared voice outcomes after Wendler glottoplasty with and without voice therapy showed that voice therapy was associated with higher F0, improved self-evaluation, and increased perception of feminine voice.

Surgical Interventions

Although voice therapy and behavior changes are the first step in voice transition for transgender patients, when the desired gender perception or pitch is not achieved, phonosurgery may be offered as an adjunct procedure. It is important to stress that vocal fold surgeries only result in alterations of vocal pitch through adjustments in the length, mass, and tension of the vocal cords. To be successfully perceived as a woman, even after surgery, patients must still maintain successful changes in airflow patterns, resonance or FF ranges, intonation, volume, and pragmatics of communication that are gender consistent. Although early surgical procedures used open technique, more recent literature favors endoscopic methods.

Open procedures allow for alteration of the laryngeal framework. In 1983, Isshiki and colleagues[18] proposed the use of cricothyroid approximation (CTA) to elevate pitch. By inferiorly displacing the larynx and suturing the thyroid ala to the cricoid, the vocal folds are stretched as if mimicking cricothyroid muscle contraction. However, subsequent studies show that pitch drops over time after CTA.[19] Thomas and Mcmillan[20] also described an open and laryngoplasty, titled FemLar (feminization laryngoplasty), that removes the anterior third of the thyroid cartilage, vocal folds, and false folds to create a new anterior commissure and promote a more feminine pitch. The average speaking pitch after this procedure increased from 139 Hz to 196 Hz.

Endoscopic approaches focus more on altering the vocal folds rather than the laryngeal framework. Many techniques describe creating an anterior web in order to shorten the vocal folds and create more tension. The CO_2 laser has also been proposed as a tool to alter the mass of the vocal folds.

Anderson[21] proposed the formation of an anterior glottic web by endoscopically removing the anterior 40% to 50% of epithelium using curved microscissors and medializing the anterior vocal fold with Radiesse Voice Gel to promote web formation. F0 increased from a preoperative mean of 127 (range 96–155) Hz to postoperative mean of 238 (range 169–360) Hz.

The CO_2 laser has also been used to alter the vocal folds. Orloff and colleagues[22] proposed using the CO_2 laser to stiffen the vocal folds to decrease their mass and increase tension, thus increasing pitch. Vaporization is made along the superior edge just 1 to 2 mm lateral from the medial edge. Mean F0 increased from 142 Hz to 168 Hz, but 3 of the 18 patients demonstrated a decrease in F0. Geneid and colleagues[23] proposed a combination of techniques by first creating a raw surface on the anterior medial mucosal edge and suturing the mucosa but not including the vocal ligament. Once this is complete, a deep longitudinal CO_2 laser cordotomy is made to the level of the muscle. Mean fundamental frequency increased from 157 to 207 Hz.

Wendler described suturing the anterior portion of the vocal folds together. Wendler glottoplasty consists of ablation of the anterior vocal fold epithelium and suturing the 2 ligaments with or without final application of fibrin glue. The suture is pulled through the muscle in order to shorten the functional length of the vocal fold (see **Fig. 1**). Healing can take several weeks, and functional outcomes improve with adjunct voice therapy (**Fig. 2**). One group reported an increase in F0 from 136 Hz to 206 Hz.[24] In another study, patients on average increased F0 from 136 Hz to 229 Hz after undergoing Wendler glottoplasty.[25] Because many MtF patients are misperceived on the telephone, 1 study used the telephone test as a tool to measure outcomes after Wendler glottoplasty.[16] There was a correlation between F0 and being perceived as a woman. However, despite achieving a higher F0, some MtF patients were still perceived as a man. One possible reason for being misgendered is the inability of the patients to maintain other changes in communication that influence gender perception.

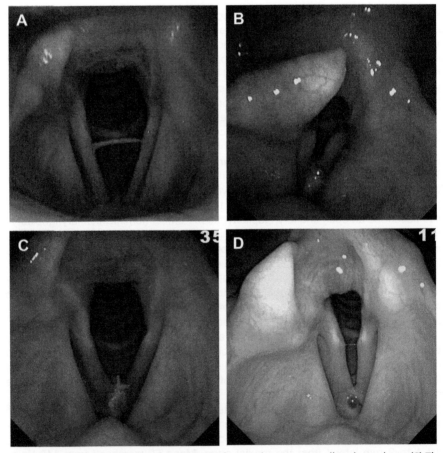

Fig. 2. (*A*) Office laryngoscopy of a patient before undergoing Wendler glottoplasty. (*B*) The same patient 1 week after Wendler glottoplasty. (*C*) Suture remnants are still visible at 1 month after surgery. (*D*) At 3 months, the larynx is almost completely healed with only a small asymptomatic granuloma. (*Courtesy of* M. S. Courey, MD, New York, NY.)

Therefore, before proceeding with surgical intervention, the importance of these other changes in communication styles for successful transition must be stressed, because there was a correlation between being perceived as a woman on the telephone and patient satisfaction with their voice and surgical outcome.

In the largest cohort of feminization phonosurgery, Kim[26] described a similar technique that deepithelializes the anterior one-third to one-half of the vocal folds and reapproximates the membranous vocal folds by suturing the lateral thyroarytenoid and vocalis muscles in 2 layers. All patients participated in voice therapy after surgery, and some were offered botulinum toxin injections to alleviate strain. The 362 patients included in the study demonstrated an average increase in pitch from 144 Hz to 207 Hz. Results from this study noted that younger patients had greater increase in pitch than older patients. Also, those who had previously received thyroid cartilage reduction, or shaving the thyroid cartilage prominence, experienced less improvement in F0 than those who did not receive thyroid cartilage reduction.

In general, the reported results for voice feminization surgery are overwhelmingly positive, but many studies are case series and retrospective reviews of a single technique.[27] A meta-analysis published in 2017 found that endoscopic techniques that shortened vocal folds were associated with the largest increase in F0.[19] However, a separate meta-analysis published in the same year reported the current evidence is insufficient to conclude a superior surgical technique.[28] Many investigators included patient-reported outcomes and satisfaction in their published results, but until the recently validated TVQ, there were no standardized questionnaires to compare these results across studies. Future research should focus on comparing techniques with standard outcomes measures.

FEMALE-TO-MALE TRANSITION

The FtM transgender population is underrepresented in the voice literature and poses unique challenges to the treatment team.[8,13] Few studies have examined objective voice changes in the FtM transgender population, and each is limited by small sample size. Patient-reported satisfaction is correlated with lower F0.[7] However, not all FtM patients respond to androgen therapy in the same way, and there is much to explore in the process of transitioning.

Hormone Therapy

Testosterone treatment is usually the first therapy FtM patients receive in the gender reassignment process. Androgen therapy with behavioral changes is often able to create a satisfactory male voice, and surgery is rarely necessary. Androgen therapy results in muscle bulking and thickening of the pharyngeal and laryngeal tissue. The result is a natural change in pitch and FF. Patients, therefore, are freer to concentrate on behavioral therapies that adjust airflow, volume, and communication pragmatics. Androgen therapy is able to decrease F0 by 70 Hz, on average, in most patients.[7] One study found a predictive correlation between serum androgen level and self-reported voice outcome in the first 3 months of androgen therapy.[12]

Although most patients who undergo androgen therapy are able to achieve a perceivable male voice, there is a small portion of FtM patients who experience voice disorders after their transition. A cross-sectional study comparing 38 FtM patients who underwent androgen therapy and gender reassignment and 38 matched male controls found no statistically significant difference in pitch.[3] However, the study did find that FtM patients with lower-pitched voices were associated with higher hematocrit and CAG repeats in the androgen receptor gene. Results of this study suggest that individual response to androgen therapy may be different because of the sensitivity of the receptor gene.

Voice Therapy

A common misconception is that androgen therapy will effectively change the voice for all FtM patients. Despite the changes in F0, some FtM patients also require voice therapy for a successful transition.[13] In the study by Nygren and colleagues[7] of 50 FtM patients, 12 (24%) patients required voice therapy at some point after starting androgen treatment. Voice therapy can help patients achieve the most efficient voice output and produce the pitch variation, intensity, and quality that is associated with a masculine voice. Furthermore, transgender patients are exposed to the same factors or practices that compromise voice function as their cisgender counterparts (for example, muscle tension can cause a strained voice and inefficient overuse can cause nodules).[8]

One review noted that some FtM patients undergo self-guided changes without involving assistance from voice professionals.[8] This practice could lead to the use of excessive muscle tension to produce a more satisfactory voice at the detriment of voice function. Other practices used by some FtM patients in order to change their voice include increasing smoking and alcohol consumption, chest-binding, and posture changes.[8] These practices may compromise voice in other ways and further illustrate the need to extend voice therapy services to this population.

Surgical Interventions

Few cases of surgical intervention have been described to lower pitch in FtM transgender patients. The most common procedure described is a type 3 thyroplasty to relax and shorten the vocal folds.[13,29] First described in 1974 by Isshiki and colleagues,[30] the procedure entails partial resection of the thyroid cartilage that relaxes the tension of the vocal folds and decreases pitch.

SUMMARY

Voice is a key component of transition for the transgender patient. It is confirmation of self-identification as well as gender perceived by others. A multidisciplinary team is often needed to appropriately manage patients' expectations and guide their progress. Voice therapy and behavioral changes are fundamental and critical for optimal outcomes. Phonosurgery should be offered as an adjunct for the appropriate patient in order to alter pitch by changing the tension, length, and mass of the vocal folds. Future directions of research should be 2 prong: to rigorously study the most efficient and effective management for MtF and FtM transgender patients and to address gaps in treatment of those who are at risk of developing voice disorders during and after their transition process.

REFERENCES

1. Winter S, Diamond M, Green J, et al. Transgender people: health at the margins of society. Lancet 2016;388(10042):390–400.
2. Hancock AB, Garabedian LM. Transgender voice and communication treatment: a retrospective chart review of 25 cases. Int J Lang Commun Disord 2013;48(1): 54–65.
3. Cosyns M, Van Borsel J, Wierckx K, et al. Voice in female-to-male transsexual persons after long-term androgen therapy. Laryngoscope 2014;124(6):1409–14.

4. Gelfer MP, Tice RM. Perceptual and acoustic outcomes of voice therapy for male-to-female transgender individuals immediately after therapy and 15 months later. J Voice 2013;27(3):335–47.

5. Neumann K, Welzel C. The importance of the voice in male-to-female transsexualism. J Voice 2004;18(1):153–67.

6. Gelfer MP, Schofield KJ. Comparison of acoustic and perceptual measures of voice in male-to-female transsexuals perceived as female versus those perceived as male. J Voice 2000;14(1):22–33.

7. Nygren U, Nordenskjold A, Arver S, et al. Effects on voice fundamental frequency and satisfaction with voice in trans men during testosterone treatment-a longitudinal study. J Voice 2016;30(6):766.e23-34.

8. Azul D, Nygren U, Sodersten M, et al. Transmasculine people's voice function: a review of the currently available evidence. J Voice 2017;31(2):261.e9-23.

9. Hancock A, Colton L, Douglas F. Intonation and gender perception: applications for transgender speakers. J Voice 2014;28(2):203–9.

10. Dacakis G, Davies S, Oates JM, et al. Development and preliminary evaluation of the transsexual voice questionnaire for male-to-female transsexuals. J Voice 2013;27(3):312–20.

11. Dacakis G, Oates JM, Douglas JM. Further evidence of the construct validity of the transsexual voice questionnaire (TVQ(MtF)) using principal components analysis. J Voice 2017;31(2):142–8.

12. Bultynck C, Pas C, Defreyne J, et al. Self-perception of voice in transgender persons during cross-sex hormone therapy. Laryngoscope 2017;127(12):2796–804.

13. Azul D. Transmasculine people's vocal situations: a critical review of gender-related discourses and empirical data. Int J Lang Commun Disord 2015;50(1): 31–47.

14. Gorham-Rowan M, Morris R. Aerodynamic analysis of male-to-female transgender voice. J Voice 2006;20(2):251–62.

15. Carew L, Dacakis G, Oates J. The effectiveness of oral resonance therapy on the perception of femininity of voice in male-to-female transsexuals. J Voice 2007; 21(5):591–603.

16. Meister J, Kuhn H, Shehata-Dieler W, et al. Perceptual analysis of the male-to-female transgender voice after glottoplasty—the telephone test. Laryngoscope 2017;127(4):875–81.

17. Gallena SJK, Stickels B, Stickels E. Gender perception after raising vowel fundamental and formant frequencies: considerations for oral resonance research. J Voice 2018;32(5):592–601.

18. Isshiki N, Taira T, Tanabe M. Surgical alteration of the vocal pitch. J Otolaryngol 1983;12(5):335–40.

19. Song TE, Jiang N. Transgender phonosurgery: a systematic review and meta-analysis. Otolaryngol Head Neck Surg 2017;156(5):803–8.

20. Thomas JP, Macmillan C. Feminization laryngoplasty: assessment of surgical pitch elevation. Eur Arch Otorhinolaryngol 2013;270(10):2695–700.

21. Anderson JA. Pitch elevation in trangendered patients: anterior glottic web formation assisted by temporary injection augmentation. J Voice 2014;28(6):816–21.

22. Orloff LA, Mann AP, Damrose JF, et al. Laser-assisted voice adjustment (LAVA) in transsexuals. Laryngoscope 2006;116(4):655–60.

23. Geneid A, Rihkanen H, Kinnari TJ. Long-term outcome of endoscopic shortening and stiffening of the vocal folds to raise the pitch. Eur Arch Otorhinolaryngol 2015; 272(12):3751–6.

24. Mastronikolis NS, Remacle M, Biagini M, et al. Wendler glottoplasty: an effective pitch raising surgery in male-to-female transsexuals. J Voice 2013;27(4):516–22.
25. Casado JC, Rodriguez-Parra MJ, Adrian JA. Voice feminization in male-to-female transgendered clients after Wendler's glottoplasty with vs. without voice therapy support. Eur Arch Otorhinolaryngol 2017;274(4):2049–58.
26. Kim HT. A new conceptual approach for voice feminization: 12 years of experience. Laryngoscope 2017;127(5):1102–8.
27. Van Damme S, Cosyns M, Deman S, et al. The effectiveness of pitch-raising surgery in male-to-female transsexuals: a systematic review. J Voice 2017;31(2): 244.e1-5.
28. Schwarz K, Fontanari AMV, Schneider MA, et al. Laryngeal surgical treatment in transgender women: a systematic review and meta-analysis. Laryngoscope 2017;127(11):2596–603.
29. Saito Y, Nakamura K, Itani S, et al. Type 3 thyroplasty for a patient with female-to-male gender identity disorder. Case Rep Otolaryngol 2018;2018:4280381.
30. Isshiki N, Morita H, Okamura H, et al. Thyroplasty as a new phonosurgical technique. Acta Otolaryngol 1974;78(5–6):451–7.

Reflux and the Voice
Getting Smarter About Laryngopharyngeal Reflux

Thomas L. Carroll, MD[a,b],*

KEYWORDS

- Laryngopharyngeal reflux • Dysphonia • Multichannel intraluminal impedance testing
- GERD • LPR • Extraesophageal reflux • EER • Atypical reflux

KEY POINTS

- Dysphonia, like other nonspecific laryngeal complaints, may be caused by LPR; however, jumping to the conclusion that LPR is the sole cause of a patient's symptoms is often naive.
- Laryngovideostroboscopy must be implemented in the face of a patient with a dysphonic complaint to determine if structural or neurologic changes are present within the glottis.
- Vocal fold pathology can be treated first in an effort to determine what LPR-like symptoms are due to vocal fold/compensatory laryngeal pathology and which symptoms are due to an underlying inflammatory problem.
- In the face of dysphonia and if no pathology beyond classic LPR signs are seen in the laryngopharynx after stroboscopy is performed then objective reflux testing is indicated.
- High-resolution manometry and hypopharyngeal-esophageal multichannel intraluminal impedance with dual pH testing should be offered if available and the patient is agreeable.

INTRODUCTION

Reflux is a general term to describe the retrograde flow of gastric contents into the structures above the stomach. Refluxate can be acidic (pH <4), weakly acidic (pH 4–7), or nonacidic (pH >7). Gastroesophageal reflux disease (GERD) is the retrograde flow of stomach contents into the esophagus causing classic symptoms such as heartburn, regurgitation, or epigastric discomfort among others. Laryngopharyngeal reflux (LPR), also known as extraesophageal reflux or atypical reflux, is the retrograde

Disclosure Statement: Sofregen Medical, Inc. Scientific Advisory board, Shareholder, Patent. Dr T.L. Carroll is a Consultant at Pentax Medical Inc.

[a] Department of Otolaryngology–Head and Neck Surgery, Harvard Medical School, Boston, MA, USA; [b] Brigham and Women's Voice Program, Division of Otolaryngology, Brigham and Women's Hospital, 45 Francis Street, Boston, MA 02115, USA
* Corresponding author. Division of Otolaryngology, 45 Francis Street, Boston, MA 02115.
E-mail address: tcarroll@bwh.harvard.edu

Otolaryngol Clin N Am 52 (2019) 723–733
https://doi.org/10.1016/j.otc.2019.03.015
0030-6665/19/© 2019 Elsevier Inc. All rights reserved.

oto.theclinics.com

flow of stomach contents into the upper esophageal sphincter and laryngopharynx and must be approached, evaluated, and treated differently than GERD. When symptomatic, LPR is called LPR disease (LPRD).[1] LPRD and GERD can coexist; however, it is not uncommon for patients with LPR to deny they have reflux due to the absence of typical GERD symptoms and for patients with GERD to never be diagnosed by an otolaryngologist for common throat symptoms that may be due to underling reflux in the setting of symptoms commonly blamed on allergies, sinonasal disease, and asthma. Depending on the prior course of treatment and the types of physicians the patient has encountered previously, the LPR-knowledgeable physician may have to re-educate and spend more time changing prior patient perceptions based on previous treatments and ineffective outcomes.

LPR remains primarily (and unfortunately) a diagnosis of exclusion in most clinical settings. LPR therefore remains misdiagnosed and overdiagnosed as the cause of many laryngeal complaints.[2] Patients with a variety of laryngeal disorders can present with identical, vague throat symptoms including globus sensation, throat clearing, mucous sensation, postnasal drip, chronic cough, laryngeal disordered breathing complaints (ie, paradoxic vocal fold motion [PVFM]), and dysphonia, none of which are truly specific to LPR.[3,4] Despite LPR being implicated as the cause of a myriad of nonspecific pharyngeal symptoms, LPR as a physiologic process is common. Whether or not it is a contributor to a patient's symptoms, especially dysphonia, is the focus of this article.

BACKGROUND
Pepsin

The primary mediator of the effects that reflux has on the laryngopharyngeal mucosa is pepsin, a proteolytic enzyme and a derivative of the proenzyme pepsinogen, which is secreted by the gastric chief cells and broken down to pepsin in an acidic environment from hydrochloric acid secreted from the gastric parietal cells.[5] Although the stomach and esophagus have some native protection against pepsin, the upper aerodigestive tract does not.[6] Pepsin is implicated in laryngopharyngeal mucosal pathology with resultant LPR signs and symptoms.[7] Pepsin has also been demonstrated to cause a release of intracellular inflammatory mediators at neutral pH.[8] The presence of pepsin correlated better with resolution of LPR-specific symptoms in patients with both LPR and GERD complaints who underwent fundoplication.[9] Moderating the deposition of pepsin seems to be a better target for diagnostic and therapeutic modalities. Despite recommendations by the American Gastroenterological Association against the empirical use of proton pump inhibitors (PPIs) for the treatment of LPR symptoms in the absence of GERD, widespread empirical PPI therapy is still a first-line treatment for LPR (with or without laryngoscopy depending on who the patient is seeing). This has significant negative implications in the use of health care dollars in the United States.

Cost and Proton Pump Inhibitor Safety

Driving forces of cost containment and patient safety are pushing otolaryngologists to better understand, diagnose, and ultimately treat LPR more effectively.[10,11] PPIs are also emerging as a medication that physicians and their patients are not eager to use due to increased concern for their association with a variety of adverse effects. Recent evidence has linked PPI use to renal disease, *Clostridium difficile* colitis, and dementia among others.[12–16] Although these types of associations are typically thought to be an issue with long-term PPI use, the negative media attention garnered by such studies influence patients' willingness to take PPIs without a clear indication; alternatives to the empirical trial approach are needed.

NEW PATIENT EVALUATION

When a patient presents with a history that includes dysphonia, but also suggests possible LPR, it is important to keep an open mind and not blame the dysphonia on LPR alone.

History

A thorough history is more important in the author's experience than the findings of the flexible laryngoscopic examination (without stroboscopy) in most cases of suspect LPR. A few key historical elements are worth emphasizing and may help the treating clinician lean toward or away from LPR contributing to the patient's problem (**Box 1**).

Box 1
Important patient history considerations for suspected laryngopharyngeal reflux

- Increased morning LPR complaints including dysphonia implicates LPR as a contributing problem; alternatively, worsening dysphonia as the day goes on can indicate a primary voice disorder, with secondary muscle tension leading to fatigue through increased effort.

- A history of postnasal drip in the absence of other rhinologic or allergic complaints and with a normal nasal examination may implicate LPR rather than allergic rhinitis.

- Classic LPR symptoms such as chronic cough, throat clearing, and mucous sensation may represent underlying glottic insufficiency and not only LPR.[3,4]

- LPR symptoms in the face of gastroesophageal reflux disease (GERD) where the patient tastes reflux events routinely may be enough to move to empirical treatments beyond what has been tried previously in that patient rather than test further. If this is not successful, multichannel intraluminal impedance with dual pH testing on reflux medications should be offered to determine why a patient is failing to relieve their symptoms. At the very least, screening esophageal endoscopy should be performed.

- Patients with histories that suggest PVFM require a workup for underlying LPR, especially nonacid LPR (in the author's experience, nonacid LPR is commonly the missing link in this group and ruling it in/out early is helpful).[17]

- A sudden voice change in the setting of a cough, sneeze, scream, or prolonged talking over loud noise with subsequent throat clearing, dysphonia, and globus should suggest acute true vocal fold pathology such as hemorrhage or hemorrhagic polyp; and like any dysphonic complaint, LVS should be included in the evaluation if the cause of the acute change is not evident on plain flexible laryngoscopy.

- Because most LPR events occur in the daytime while upright, patients must be educated to understand why their symptoms may be reflux related without feeling GERD or night-time symptoms.

- Adult patients with a diagnosis of asthma and LPR complaints should be given special consideration. Many asthma patients have never had testing to rule in or rule out asthma (pulmonary function testing with bronchodilator challenge; methacholine challenge etc.) and have been put on steroid inhalers empirically. A thorough evaluation of their prior workup is often revealing.[18]

- Postviral vagal neuropathy (PVVN) typically occurs after an otherwise routine viral illness and can understandably lead to a host of LPR-associated complaints that often affect the aerodigestive tract due to the distribution of the vagus nerve including the recurrent laryngeal nerve.[19] PVVN can lead to disorders of esophageal and gastric motility and esophageal sphincter dysfunction; the dysfunction of involuntary muscles involved with reflux protection and peristalsis can allow new, real LPR.[20]

Reflux Symptom Index

The reflux symptom index (RSI) is a 9-item questionnaire developed by Belafsky and colleagues[21] using pH-only testing without impedance to determine if LPR is present (**Fig. 1**). Anecdotally in practice, the RSI seems less useful for diagnosing LPR but rather a good tool for following vague throat symptoms over time regardless of the cause.[22] Small studies have made the connection between LPR-attributed symptoms and glottic insufficiency and at least one study has demonstrated that the optimal RSI cutoff may be different in patients with concomitant allergic disease.[3,4,23]

EXAMINATION

Dysphonia in any setting warrants laryngoscopy within 4 weeks of symptom onset, possibly sooner in certain situations such as the patient being a smoker.[24]

Reflux Finding Score

The reflux finding score (RFS) is an 8-item rating scale derived by Belafsky and colleagues[25] to facilitate a standardized approach to assessing LPR using physical findings on flexible laryngoscopy without stroboscopy in patients with pH, but not impedance proven, LPR. Unfortunately, laryngeal findings attributed to reflux and documented using the RFS may also be seen in healthy volunteers.[25–27] More recent data cast a shadow on the reliability of the RFS.[28–30]

Laryngovideostroboscopy

In the setting of dysphonia and a normal flexible laryngoscopic examination, laryngovideostroboscopy (LVS) is required to truly diagnose the cause of the patient's

RSI- Instructions: These are statements that many people have used to describe their voices and the effects of their voices on their lives. Circle the response that indicates how frequently you have the same experience.

Within the last MONTH, how did the following problems affect you?

0 = No problem   5 = Severe Problem

Hoarseness or a problem with your voice	0	1	2	3	4	5
Clearing your throat	0	1	2	3	4	5
Excess throat mucous	0	1	2	3	4	5
Difficulty swallowing food, liquids or pills	0	1	2	3	4	5
Coughing after eating or after lying down	0	1	2	3	4	5
Breathing difficulties or choking episodes	0	1	2	3	4	5
Troublesome or annoying cough	0	1	2	3	4	5
Sensations of something sticking in your throat or a lump in your throat	0	1	2	3	4	5
Heartburn, chest pain, indigestion, or stomach acid coming up	0	1	2	3	4	5

Fig. 1. Reflux symptom index. (*Adapted from* Belafsky PC, Postma GN, Koufman JA, et al. Validity and reliability of the reflux symptom index (RSI). J Voice 2002;16(2):275; with permission.)

hoarseness by assessing mucosal wave and glottic closure pattern. LVS may reveal subtle true vocal fold (TVF) lesions, scar, or subtle atrophy/paresis with air escape during phonation (glottic insufficiency).[24] Although LVS is not required (routinely) to rule out cancer, most patients, while glad they do not have "throat cancer," want to know why they are dysphonic and LVS is needed in most situations.

Two outcomes are possible from the LVS examination: a finding that explains the patient's dysphonic complaint or no clear TVF or glottic closure finding to explain the symptoms. If the former, reflux may remain on the table but it may also be worthwhile to treat the laryngeal pathology with the help of a speech-language pathologist or procedural/surgical intervention to see what symptoms improve before exploring LPR further. Glottic insufficiency is often present in the face of supraglottic hyperfunction (with intrinsic and extrinsic laryngeal muscle compensatory behaviors) although functional voice and swallowing disorders are real but less common in the author's experience.[31–35]

OBJECTIVE TESTING FOR REFLUX
Transnasal Esophagoscopy and Esophagogastroduodenoscopy

Transnasal esophagoscopy (TNE) uses a sub-6 mm flexible endoscope to evaluate the esophagus in the awake clinical setting. It can be performed relatively quickly in an office setting, most often by laryngologists and has proved to be as effective and reliable as esophagogastroduodenoscopy (EGD).[36] TNE seems to be more valuable as a screening tool in patients already known to have LPR rather than as a tool in the diagnosis and workup of LPR.[37–39]

EGD is used to evaluate the esophagus, stomach, and proximal portion of the duodenum. It is typically performed by gastroenterologists using a 10-mm flexible endoscope with the patient under sedation for suspected reflux. A positive esophageal screening with pathologic diagnostic biopsies can reveal evidence of reflux including esophagitis, ulceration, as well as longer-term sequelae such as stricture formation and the premalignant finding of Barrett's esophagus. It is important to remember that a normal EGD does not rule out reflux as the cause of LPR symptoms.

Manometry

High-resolution esophageal manometry (HRM) is a necessary adjunct in the workup of LPR-suspect patients. HRM is a catheter-based test that determines the ability of the esophageal muscles to contract and move the bolus through in a coordinated fashion. It can identify the upper and lower esophageal sphincters (UES and LES) and thus afford correct placement of the upper pH probe of the hypopharyngeal-esophageal multichannel intraluminal impedance with dual pH (HEMII-pH) catheter. HRM can identify a hiatal hernia as well as esophageal dysmotility that may contribute to a patient's LPR symptoms.[40,41]

Measuring pH in Pharynx

Direct pharyngeal pH measurement is popular among otolaryngologists due to ease of placement, better tolerance by patients, and convenient scoring of results.[42] Despite its ability to detect a range of pH and not just acid, the Restech probe (Respiratory Technology Corporation, Houston, TX, USA) was not able to reliably differentiate between healthy volunteers and subjects with a combination of laryngeal and reflux symptoms, nor could it predict response to PPI therapy.[43,44] In addition, as when both HEMII-pH and Restech were used simultaneously, it was determined that Restech was not detecting true LPR events as seen on HEMII-pH.[45]

Hypopharyngeal-Esophageal Impedance with Dual pH Testing

HEMII-pH testing is the new gold standard for LPR diagnosis. Multichannel intraluminal impedance and pH (MII-pH) catheters allow for acid and nonacid reflux detection up to the proximal esophagus (15–17 cm above LES). Impedance sensors measure electrical resistance between an electrode pair. When these electrode pairs are placed along a catheter, as is done with impedance testing for reflux, detection of both gaseous and liquid reflux episodes, as well as their direction of flow over time, are reported regardless of acidity. With the addition of 2 pH sensors, one distal and one proximal (to be placed at or above the UES), HEMII-pH testing can now provide the number and extent of acidic and nonacidic reflux episodes throughout and beyond the esophageal column into the hypopharynx over a 24-hour period.[46,47] The patient undergoes HRM from which the location of the UES is determined and the HEMII-pH catheter is then placed and taped to the patient's cheek and further attached to a recording device. It is worn by the patient for up to 24 hours. The patient can also press one of 3 buttons on the recording device to report an LPR or GERD symptom to determine if what they experience coordinates with an actual reflux event.

Hypopharyngeal-Esophageal Impedance-pH Interpretation

Normative studies of HEMII-pH using healthy controls have shown that as few as 2 reflux events (either acid or nonacid) reaching the pharynx in a 24-hour period may be considered abnormal.[48,49] In contrast, it may be normal for as many as 31 reflux events (acid or nonacid) to reach the proximal esophagus in the same amount of time.[46] Borges and colleagues[46] demonstrated this using previous criteria for abnormal numbers of impedance events in the distal esophagus and at 17 cm above the LES. They showed that older technology and GERD-centric interpretation may not be able to predict LPR events. Pharyngeal reflux detection has shown promise in the workup of extraesophageal manifestations of reflux in patients with both adult-onset asthma and idiopathic pulmonary fibrosis, 2 lung diseases in which extraesophageal reflux is postulated to play a role.[50,51]

Whether or not 2 pharyngeal events are enough to be the causative agent of a patient's LPR symptoms remains incompletely understood. However, studies using HEMII-pH are emerging that demonstrate resolution of LPR symptoms after antireflux surgery.[48] The combination of pharyngeal and esophageal pH-impedance testing is far from a conclusive test in many situations. A study by Dulery and colleagues[52] concluded that combined esophageal and pharyngeal pH-impedance testing may have limited utility in patients with LPR symptoms refractory to PPI therapy because the subjects did not have significant pharyngeal impedance events. The Dulery study highlights 2 important aspects of HEMII-pH testing. First, interpretation of pharyngeal impedance events is variable, even between physician experts (low intrarater reliability), and second, high esophageal (aka at the UES but not across) may need closer evaluation as the more reliable marker when interpreting HEMII-pH testing, as pharyngeal events can be skewed by swallows.[49] HEMII-pH testing currently provides the most in-depth assessment of a patient's reflux burden when compared with other testing modalities. This is despite a solid, but incomplete, understanding of the pathophysiology of why some patients with few pharyngeal events are very symptomatic and others with many events are less so.

Salivary Pepsin Assays

Salivary pepsin rapid detection assays are available, not widely so in the United States. There is evidence that finding pepsin in saliva is 78% sensitive and 65%

specific for the diagnosis of LPR, with increased specificity in the setting of higher pepsin concentrations.[53] However, a small study of 35 subjects was unable to differentiate between healthy controls and subjects with LPR signs and symptoms using salivary pepsin.[43] A 2017 systematic review on available salivary pepsin literature concluded that many questions remain about pepsin testing in the face of an LPR-suspect patient.[54] Salivary pepsin testing shows correlation with reflux diagnosed with nonpharyngeal MII-pH catheters and may prove itself as an adjunct test in the workup of LPR but currently remains limited in its use.

TREATMENTS

Empirical acid suppression remains a popular treatment and diagnostic tool for LPR suspect patients. However, as this article has emphasized, empirical PPI trials may not be the safest or most cost-effective option. If objective testing demonstrates acid reflux or if an empirical trial is warranted, starting with a once daily high-dose PPI (ie, omeprazole, 40 mg) in the morning and a bedtime dose of high-dose H2 blocker (ie, ranitidine, 300 mg) is a reasonable starting regimen with elevation to 40 mg PPI twice a day for nonresponders after 3 months.[11] If the patient does not respond to the high-dose BID PPI then it must be realized that nonacid reflux has not been ruled out and HEMII-pH testing is indicated if it can be obtained.

Treating Nonacid Reflux

Every patient suspected or diagnosed with LPR should be educated about the pathophysiology of pepsin-mediated LPR and offered diet and lifestyle changes. Typically, these changes include instructions for classic GERD such as head of bed elevation, not eating close to bedtime, less spicy food, less alcohol, weight loss etc. LPR may not really need these and a diet lower in acidic food may make more sense.[55] Pepsin is most active in low pH so when pharyngeal pepsin is exposed to an acid environment, whether from oral intake or gastric reflux, the pepsin will cause inflammation regardless of the source. Many patients who make dramatic changes in their diet notice improvement in their LPR symptoms; however most people cannot follow such a strict regimen. Alkaline water consumption may denature pepsin in the pharynx and thus may be a nonharmful and likely helpful adjunct to diet and lifestyle changes.[56]

Forming a barrier to LPR in the stomach is a crucial part of the treatment of LPR. Nissen fundoplication (Nissen) can be recommended to anyone with proven LPR; however, most patients without significantly debilitating symptoms elect to undergo this procedure. The success of Nissen in relieving LPR symptoms in patients selected using HEMII-pH testing looks promising.[48] For patients who need a barrier but do not want Nissen or may not tolerate it (poor esophageal motility etc.), alginate agents are a great option. Alginates are derived from seaweed and are sold as chewable tablets or as a liquid suspension mixed with salts (ie, Gaviscon Advance, Reckitt-Benckiser, Slough, United Kingdom). Different countries in the world sell different versions of "Gaviscon." Each dose of alginate should include approximately 1000 mg of the alginate itself. Gaviscon Advance from the UK has this in 10 mL of suspension and the Canadian version, Gaviscon Max Relief (Prestige Brands, Inc., Canada) provides this amount in 3 chewable tablets. The version in the United States has much less alginate, includes aluminum, and requires a less tolerable amount of liquid per dose.

SUMMARY

LPR is too often implicated in the workup of dysphonia. Dysphonia, like other nonspecific laryngeal complaints may be caused by LPR; however, jumping to the conclusion that LPR is the sole cause of a patient's symptoms is often naive. Laryngovideostroboscopy must be implemented in the face of a patient with a dysphonic complaint to determine if structural or neurologic changes are present within the glottis. If no pathologic conditions beyond classic LPR signs are seen in the laryngopharynx, high-resolution manometry and HEMII-pH testing should be offered if available and the patient is agreeable. Despite treating vocal fold pathology, LPR may be a concomitant problem and may have been an underlying source of inflammation that leads to true vocal fold lesion formation. The astute clinician who treats dysphonic patients must be flexible in their approach and consider LPR when appropriate while at the same time not blaming LPR for all unexplained laryngeal complaints. Once diagnosed as a contributor to symptoms, diet, lifestyle, and barrier treatments can be offered.

REFERENCES

1. Ford CN. Evaluation and management of laryngopharyngeal reflux. JAMA 2005; 294(12):1534–40.
2. Cohen SM, Garrett CG. Hoarseness: is it really laryngopharyngeal reflux? Laryngoscope 2008;118(2):363–6.
3. Crawley BK, Murry T, Sulica L. Injection augmentation for chronic cough. J Voice 2015;29(6):763–7.
4. Patel AK, Mildenhall NR, Kim W, et al. Symptom overlap between laryngopharyngeal reflux and glottic insufficiency in vocal fold atrophy patients. Ann Otol Rhinol Laryngol 2014;123(4):265–70.
5. Johnston N, Dettmar PW, Bishwokarma B, et al. Activity/stability of human pepsin: implications for reflux attributed laryngeal disease. Laryngoscope 2007;117(6): 1036–9.
6. Johnston N, Dettmar PW, Strugala V, et al. Laryngopharyngeal reflux and GERD. Ann N Y Acad Sci 2013;1300:71–9.
7. Adhami T, Goldblum JR, Richter JE, et al. The role of gastric and duodenal agents in laryngeal injury: an experimental canine model. Am J Gastroenterol 2004;99: 2098–106.
8. Johnston N, Wells CW, Blumin JH, et al. Receptor-mediated uptake of pepsin by laryngeal epithelial cells. Ann Otol Rhinol Laryngol 2007;116(12):934–8.
9. Wassenaar E, Johnston N, Merati A, et al. Pepsin detection in patients with laryngopharyngeal reflux before and after fundoplication. Surg Endosc 2011; 25(12):3870–6.
10. Francis DO, Rymer JA, Slaughter JC, et al. High economic burden of caring for patients with suspected extraesophageal reflux. Am J Gastroenterol 2013; 108(6):905.
11. Carroll TL, Werner A, Nahikian K, et al. Rethinking the laryngopharyngeal reflux treatment algorithm: evaluating an alternate empiric dosing regimen and considering up-front, pH-impedance, and manometry testing to minimize cost in treating suspect laryngopharyngeal reflux disease. Laryngoscope 2017;127:S1–13.
12. Klepser DG, Collier DS, Cochran GL. Proton pump inhibitors and acute kidney injury: a nested case-control study. BMC Nephrol 2013;14:150.
13. Kwok CS, Arthur AK, Anibueze CI, et al. Risk of Clostridium difficile infection with acid suppressing drugs and antibiotics: meta-analysis. Am J Gastroenterol 2012; 107(7):1011–9.
14. McDonald EG, Milligan J, Frenette C, et al. Continuous proton pump inhibitor therapy and the associated risk of recurrent clostridium difficile infection. JAMA Intern Med 2015;175(5):784–91.

15. Gomm W, von Holt K, Thomé F, et al. Association of proton pump inhibitors with risk of dementia. JAMA Neurol 2016. https://doi.org/10.1001/jamaneurol.2015.4791.

16. Blonski W, Vela MF, Castell DO. Comparison of reflux frequency during prolonged multichannel intraluminal impedance and ph monitoring on and off acid suppression therapy. J Clin Gastroenterol 2009;43(9):816.

17. Altman K. Cough and paradoxical vocal fold motion. Otolaryngol Head Neck Surg 2002;127(6):501–11.

18. Brigham EP, West NE. Diagnosis of asthma: diagnostic testing. Int Forum Allergy Rhinol 2015;5(S1):S27–30.

19. Rees CJ, Henderson AH, Belafsky PC. Postviral vagal neuropathy. Ann Otol Rhinol Laryngol 2009;118(4):247–52.

20. Martinucci I, de Bortoli N, Giacchino M, et al. Esophageal motility abnormalities in gastroesophageal reflux disease. World J Gastrointest Pharmacol Ther 2014; 5(2):86–96.

21. Belafsky PC, Postma GN, Koufman JA. Validity and reliability of the reflux symptom index (RSI). Journal of voice 2002;16(2):274–7.

22. Rosen CA, Lee AS, Osborne J, et al. Development and validation of the voice handicap index-10. Laryngoscope 2004;114(9):1549–56.

23. Brauer DL, Tse KY, Lin JC, et al. The utility of the reflux symptom index for diagnosis of laryngopharyngeal reflux in an allergy patient population. J Allergy Clin Immunol Pract 2017. https://doi.org/10.1016/j.jaip.2017.04.039.

24. Stachler RJ, Francis DO, Schwartz SR, et al. Clinical practice guideline: hoarseness (dysphonia)(update). Otolaryngol Head Neck Surg 2018;158(1_suppl): S1–42.

25. Belafsky PC, Postma GN, Koufman JA. The validity and reliability of the reflux finding score (RFS). Laryngoscope 2001;111(8):1313–7.

26. Hicks DM, Ours TM, Abelson TI, et al. The prevalence of hypopharynx findings associated with gastroesophageal reflux in normal volunteers. J Voice 2002; 16(4):564–79. Available at: http://www.ncbi.nlm.nih.gov/pubmed/12512644. Accessed July 21, 2016.

27. Milstein CF, Charbel S, Hicks DM, et al. Prevalence of laryngeal irritation signs associated with reflux in asymptomatic volunteers: impact of endoscopic technique (rigid vs. flexible laryngoscope). Laryngoscope 2005;115(12):2256–61.

28. Chang BA, MacNeil SD, Morrison MD, et al. The reliability of the reflux finding score among general otolaryngologists. J Voice 2015;29(5):572–7.

29. Wo JM, Koopman J, Harrell SP, et al. Double-blind, placebo-controlled trial with single-dose pantoprazole for laryngopharyngeal reflux. Am J Gastroenterol 2006;101(9):1972–8 [quiz: 2169].

30. Cool M, Poelmans J, Feenstra L, et al. Characteristics and clinical relevance of proximal esophageal pH monitoring. Am J Gastroenterol 2004;99(12):2317–23.

31. Altman KW, Atkinson C, Lazarus C. Current and emerging concepts in muscle tension dysphonia: a 30-month review. J Voice 2005;19(2):261–7.

32. Kang CH, Hentz JG, Lott DG. Muscle tension dysphagia symptomology and theoretical framework. Otolaryngol Head Neck Surg 2016;155(5):837–42.

33. Carroll TL, Rosen CA. Trial vocal fold injection. J Voice 2010;24(4):494–8.

34. Carroll TL, Dezube A, Bauman LA, et al. Using trial vocal fold injection to select vocal fold scar patients who may benefit from more durable augmentation. Ann Otol Rhinol Laryngol 2018;127(2):105–12.

35. Young VN, Gartner-Schmidt J, Rosen CA. Comparison of voice outcomes after trial and long-term vocal fold augmentation in vocal fold atrophy. Laryngoscope 2015;125(4):934–40.

36. Peery AF, Hoppo T, Garman KS, et al. Feasibility, safety, acceptability, and yield of office-based, screening transnasal esophagoscopy (with video). Gastrointest Endosc 2012;75(5):945–53.e2.

37. Howell RJ, Pate MB, Ishman SL, et al. Prospective multi-institutional transnasal esophagoscopy: predictors of a change in management. Laryngoscope 2016; 126(12):2667–71.

38. Madanick RD. Extraesophageal presentations of GERD. Gastroenterol Clin North Am 2014;43(1):105–20.

39. Passaretti S, Mazzoleni G, Vailati C, et al. Oropharyngeal acid reflux and motility abnormalities of the proximal esophagus. World J Gastroenterol 2016;22(40): 8991.

40. Fouad YM, Katz PO, Hatlebakk JG, et al. Ineffective esophageal motility: the most common motility abnormality in patients with GERD-associated respiratory symptoms. Am J Gastroenterol 1999;94(6):1464–7.

41. Patti MG, Debas HT, Pellegrini CA. Clinical and functional characterization of high gastroesophageal reflux. Am J Surg 1993;165(1):163–6 [discussion: 166–8]. Avialable at: http://www.ncbi.nlm.nih.gov/pubmed/8418693.

42. Chheda NN, Seybt MW, Schade RR, et al. Normal values for pharyngeal pH monitoring. Ann Otol Rhinol Laryngol 2009;118(3):166–71.

43. Yadlapati R, Adkins C, Jaiyeola D-M, et al. Abilities of oropharyngeal pH tests and salivary pepsin analysis to discriminate between asymptomatic volunteers and subjects with symptoms of laryngeal irritation. Clin Gastroenterol Hepatol 2016; 14(4):535–42.e2.

44. Yadlapati R, Pandolfino JE, Lidder AK, et al. Oropharyngeal pH testing does not predict response to proton pump inhibitor therapy in patients with laryngeal symptoms. Am J Gastroenterol 2016;111(11):1517–24.

45. Ummarino D, Vandermeulen L, Roosens B, et al. Gastroesophageal reflux evaluation in patients affected by chronic cough: restech versus multichannel intraluminal impedance/pH metry. Laryngoscope 2013;123(4):980–4.

46. Borges LF, Chan WW, Carroll TL. Dual pH probes without proximal esophageal and pharyngeal impedance may be deficient in diagnosing LPR. J Voice 2018. https://doi.org/10.1016/j.jvoice.2018.03.008.

47. Lee YC, Kwon OE, Park JM, et al. Do laryngoscopic findings reflect the characteristics of reflux in patients with laryngopharyngeal reflux? Clin Otolaryngol 2017. https://doi.org/10.1111/coa.12914.

48. Hoppo T, Komatsu Y, Jobe BA. Antireflux surgery in patients with chronic cough and abnormal proximal exposure as measured by hypopharyngeal multichannel intraluminal impedance. JAMA Surg 2013;148(7):608.

49. Zerbib F, Roman S, Bruley Des Varannes S, et al. Normal values of pharyngeal and esophageal 24-hour pH impedance in individuals on and off therapy and interobserver reproducibility. Clin Gastroenterol Hepatol 2013;11(4):366–72.

50. Hoppo T, Komatsu Y, Jobe BA. Gastroesophageal reflux disease and patterns of reflux in patients with idiopathic pulmonary fibrosis using hypopharyngeal multichannel intraluminal impedance. Dis Esophagus 2014;27(6):530–7.

51. Komatsu Y, Hoppo T, Jobe BA. Proximal reflux as a cause of adult-onset asthma. JAMA Surg 2013;148(1):50.

52. Dulery C, Lechot A, Roman S, et al. A study with pharyngeal and esophageal 24-hour pH-impedance monitoring in patients with laryngopharyngeal symptoms refractory to proton pump inhibitors. Neurogastroenterol Motil 2017;29(1):e12909.
53. Hayat JO, Gabieta-Somnez S, Yazaki E, et al. Pepsin in saliva for the diagnosis of gastro-oesophageal reflux disease. Gut 2015;64(3):373–80.
54. Calvo-Henríquez C, Ruano-Ravina A, Vaamonde P, et al. Is pepsin a reliable marker of laryngopharyngeal reflux? A systematic review. Otolaryngol Head Neck Surg 2017;157(3):385–91.
55. Koufman JA. Low-acid diet for recalcitrant laryngopharyngeal reflux: therapeutic benefits and their implications. Ann Otol Rhinol Laryngol 2011;120(5):281–7.
56. Koufman JA, Johnston N. Potential benefits of pH 8.8 alkaline drinking water as an adjunct in the treatment of reflux disease. Ann Otol Rhinol Laryngol 2012; 121(7):431–4.

Sulcus Vocalis

Resha S. Soni, MD, Seth H. Dailey, MD*

KEYWORDS

- Sulcus vocalis • Vocal fold sulcus • Sulcus vergeture • Microlaryngoscopy • Larynx
- Dysphonia

KEY POINTS

- Sulcus vocalis is an invagination of the vocal fold epithelium into the superficial lamina propria or deeper.
- Clinical presentation is characterized by dysphonia with vocal fatigue and vocal effort.
- The treatment paradigm for sulcus vocalis includes voice therapy and various open and endoscopic techniques.
- Future directions include the use of growth factors and tissue engineering.

INTRODUCTION

The vocal fold is a multilayered structure composed of an overlying stratified squamous epithelium, superficial layer of lamina propria (SLP), intermediate lamina propria, deep lamina propria, and the thyroarytenoid muscle complex. The body-cover concept of the vocal fold suggests the true vocal fold can be divided into layers with different mechanical and vibratory characteristics. The vocal fold cover consists of the epithelium and the SLP. The vocal ligament together with the underlying thyroarytenoid muscle complex make up the body.[1] The gelatinous and pliable cover is believed to move freely over the vocal fold body during voicing.[2] When the pliability of the vocal fold is compromised, glottic closure is impaired, leading to dysfunction.[3]

DEFINITION AND CLASSIFICATION

The term, *sulcus vocalis*, is used to describe a furrow running parallel to the free edge of the true vocal fold resulting in an area of decreased mucosal wave pliability.[4] The vocal fold epithelium is pathologically present in the SLP or deeper. It is a benign vocal fold anomaly of varying length and depth that results in an abnormal lamina propria configuration; the lamina propria is reduced or completely lost with subsequent poor vocal fold vibratory function.[3]

Disclosures: No commercial or financial conflicts of interest or funding to disclose.
Division of Otolaryngology–Head & Neck Surgery, Department of Surgery, University of Wisconsin Hospital and Clinics, 600 Highland Avenue, Office K4/727, Madison, WI 53792-7375, USA
* Corresponding author.
E-mail address: Dailey@surgery.wisc.edu

Otolaryngol Clin N Am 52 (2019) 735–743
https://doi.org/10.1016/j.otc.2019.03.016
0030-6665/19/© 2019 Elsevier Inc. All rights reserved.

The most commonly used description proposed by Ford and colleagues[5] classifies the severity of the lesion (**Fig. 1**):

- A type I sulcus is a depression of the epithelium into only the SLP. In general, it has limited to no functional impact and is not considered pathologic. Therefore, it is commonly referred to as a "physiologic sulcus" or a "superficial-type sulcus."
- A type II sulcus, or sulcus vergeture, is characterized by loss of the SLP with extension to the vocal ligament.
- A type III sulcus is often referred to as a "pit" or "pouch" because it is a focal indentation that extends into the vocal ligament or deeper.[6]

There is a discordance in the literature with regard to the nomenclature. Some studies using the term, sulcus vocalis, to refer only to a type III sulcus.[7] This has led to confusion and difficulty with determining prevalence. A need for a universal agreement on terminology is apparent. An important distinction should be made between sulcus vocalis and vocal fold scar, which often are grouped together in the literature. Both pathologic processes involve derangement of lamina propria resulting in abnormal vold fold viscoelastic properties. Although sulcus vocalis is characterized by a loss of lamina propria frequently accompanied by vocal fold scar, vocal fold scar itself is characterized by a deposition of abnormal, thick, fibrous tissue within the lamina propria without the necessary morphologic feature of an invaginated vocal fold surface.[8] The symptoms of patients with either are similar, including dysphonia

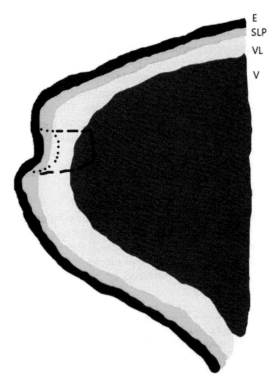

Fig. 1. Sulcus classification. Invagination of epithelium into SLP, type I sulcus (*solid black line*). Type II sulcus is invagination of epithelium into the VL (*dotted line*). Type III sulcus is invagination past the VL into the vocalis muscle (*dashed line*). E, epithelium; V, vocalis; VL, vocal ligament.

with harsh vocal quality, increased vocal fatigue, and vocal effort.[3,9,10] Sulcus vocalis and vocal fold atrophy, due to lamina propria thinning and muscle loss, also share similar characteristics.[11] The primary difference between vocal fold atrophy and sulcus vocalis is that the latter exhibit stiffness, which is not necessarily present in vocal fold atrophy.[11,12]

PATHOPHYSIOLOGY

As discussed previously, sulcus vocalis alters the physical properties of the vocal fold. There is disruption to the normal mucosal wave as a result of the varying deficiency to the vocal fold architecture.[10] It is believed that sulcus vocalis may be acquired as a result of phonotrauma to the vocal folds.[4] Histopathologic evaluation studies have demonstrated that tissues adjacent to a sulcus are found to have proliferation of fibrous tissue and blood vessels; findings that are characteristic of a chronic inflammatory process.[13] Early investigators, like Bouchayer and Cornut[6], however, speculated that this entity was congenital in nature. In their study of 157 patients, they used the following findings to support their hypothesis: early onset of dysphonia in childhood in their study population, absence of recurrence after excision, and the existence of familial cases.[6,14] In their large series of patients with sulcus vocalis, Ito and colleagues[4] noted that vocal symptoms ranged from birth to the ninth decade of life. Given that proponents for both sides have shown convincing evidence for support, it is likely that both congenital and acquired forms exist.[15]

Sato and Hirano[11] sought to deepen the understanding of changes that occur on a microscopic level. They performed electron microscopy to further study this pathologic process and noted increased thickness of the basement membrane, decreased elastic tissue, degeneration of fibroblasts in the muculae flavae—the structure responsible for ensuring synthesis of lamina propria fibrous components, and dense collagenous fibers.[11] More recently, Lee and colleagues[16] evaluated the histopathologic specimens of 15 patients with sulcus vocalis and highlighted the prominent pathologic epithelial changes not previously emphasized in other studies. They noted marked epithelial thickening, parakeratosis, and dyskeratosis, suggesting that increasing focus on this histologic layer may shift the treatment paradigm in the future.[16]

EVALUATION

Establishing a diagnosis of sulcus vocalis can prove a difficult one.[17] The patient ideally should be evaluated utilizing a multidisciplinary approach with a laryngologist and a certified speech-language pathologist trained in voice. The vocal folds may appear normal during indirect laryngoscopy so the use of videostroboscopy is an effective diagnostic tool (**Fig. 2**). Even so, Dailey and colleagues[18] retrospectively reviewed the records of 100 patients who had underdone suspension microlaryngoscopy (SML) for benign glottic lesions. Sixteen additional lesions, with the majority of these sulci, were appreciated at the time of SML, which were not previously noted during in-office evaluation with rigid stroboscopy.[18] They noted that this may be due to tangential views of the medial surface of the vocal folds during office endoscopy, which limits diagnostic ability. A more recent prospective study by Akbulut and colleagues[19] helped confirm this discrepancy between office strobopsopy and microlaryngoscopy findings. In their study, only 34% of their 85 patients had the exact same diagnosis as stroboscopy after undergoing subsequent SML. A majority of patients had an additional vocal fold structural abnormality identified, with the most common abnormality sulcus vocalis.[19]

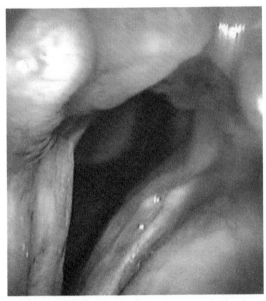

Fig. 2. Laryngeal videostroboscopy depicting left true vocal fold sulcus vocalis. Verbal and written permission obtained from patient.

Nevertheless, stroboscopy is an important in-office diagnostic tool, and the typical findings of sulcus vocalis with stroboscopy have been described: reduced amplitude of the mucosal wave, a bowed or curved aspect to the free edge of the involved vocal fold, glottic incompetence, and hyperfunction of the ventricular vocal folds in some cases from compensation.[6,10] The term, *spindle-shaped glottis*, often is used in the literature to describe the glottic closure pattern associated with sulcus vocalis; however, this is not pathognomonic and can occur with other entities.[10,20]

Other stroboscopic and aerodynamic findings also have been described. Hirano and colleagues[10] studied 126 patients with either unilateral or bilateral sulcus vocalis using a battery of vocal function tests. A majority of these patients were classified as having a type I sulcus, and they observed the following: an incomplete glottic closure, a small vibratory amplitude, decreased maximum phonation time, decreased fundamental frequency range, and increased airflow during phonation.[10]

SML is the concluding diagnostic step in the evaluation of glottic pathology. Known discordances between in-office evaluation and intraoperative findings make this step a particularly crucial one for diagnostic and therapeutic purposes. A systematic examination of the supraglottic, glottic, and subglottic subsites should be undertaken with detailed photodocumentation performed using rigid 0° and 70° telescopes. Secretions should be gently cleared and there should be meticulous palpation and evaluation of the bilateral vocal folds using a small, blunt, right-angle probe from the anterior commissure to the arytenoids.[19] Probing of the mucosal surfaces in an atraumatic fashion can display discrete structural abnormalities and better allow for classification and subsequent treatment planning.

TREATMENT OPTIONS

Historically speaking, sulcus vocalis has been hailed as a problem that is difficult to treat. As with most other benign vocal fold lesions, nonsurgical therapy should first be trialed, and then therapeutic treatment options should progress in a stepwise fashion from least invasive to maximally invasive. One should be mindful regarding the treatment of comorbid medical conditions, which may exacerbate vocal dysfunction. Reflux, active rheumatologic conditions, and sinonasal and allergic disease must be appropriately managed. A patient's functional limitations and goals should be addressed clearly, and there should be reasonable expectations with regard to vocal improvement.[18]

Studies investigating the effect of voice therapy on sulcus vocalis have shown improvement in acoustic, aerodynamic, perceptual, and Voice Handicap Index (VHI)-10 scores.[21,22] After nonsurgical intervention with voice and singing therapy has proved unsuccessful and functional limitations persist, the patient can be considered a candidate for surgical interventions. Various treatment options have been proposed, with most treatments being helpful for vocal fold scar but data on sulcus, in general, are lacking.[23]

Vocal Fold Injections

Most surgeons are familiar with an injection laryngoplasty into the paraglottic space with a variety of injection materials to improve glottic insufficiency, but this has not proved to affect the sulcus directly.[24] In-office steroid injections, to reduce the inflammation surrounding the sulcus/scar, is well described but also does not directly address the underlying extracellular matrix dysfunction.[25,26] Another technique is the injection of collagen into the sulcus/scar. Collagen, a component of the native lamina propria, can be injected into the atrophic area and is believed to aid in lamina propria remodeling.[27,28]

Medialization Thyroplasty

Initially described by Isshiki, medialization thyroplasty of the vocal fold has since been proposed with various materials (eg. Gore-Tex and strap muscle transposition).[29] As a sole modality, it does not address the sulcus directly but should be considered an adjunctive treatment to other techniques or a stand-alone technique to address glottic insufficiency.

Undermining the Sulcus

This microlaryngoscopic approach has been described with both cold instrumentation and laser techniques.[30,31] It involves a longitudinal corodotomy with release of the sulcus from its deepest attachment. This is followed by redraping of the epithelium (**Fig. 3**). An alternative to this technique is using cold instrumentation to formally excise the sulcus endoscopically. This approach is more useful for type III sulci because it understandably leaves a focal tissue defect and outcomes are not as predictable.[5] Adjunct steroid injection, fibrin glue implantation, and alloderm implantation have been best described for lesions in which the structural damage is limited. Dissection with these techniques should be performed with preservation of as much healthy tissue as possible. The belief is that subsequent wound healing will be regenerative.[26,32]

Autologous Tissue Implantation

Fat implantation into the sulcus/scar, allowing for the ability use autologous tissue and the ability to improve vocal fold pliability, make this an appealing option.[33–35] Autologous temporalis fascia implantation into the superficial vocal fold shows good long-term follow-up, high patient satisfaction, and a statistically significant decrease in VHI-10 scores.[8,36]

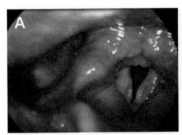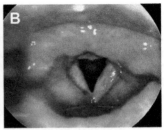

Fig. 3. (*A*) Preoperative laryngeal videostroboscopy of bilateral true vocal fold sulci. (*B*) Postoperative laryngeal videostroboscopy depicting improved bilateral sulci after cold instrumentation undermining. Patient was noted to have improved true vocal fold pliability.

Pontes Mucosal Slicing

This mucosal slicing technique as reported by Pontes and Behlau[37] exercises the principles of scar contraction in an attempt to reorganize lines of stress. An incision is initially made parallel along the vocal fold–free edge. Microinstrumentation is then used to create multiple incisions of varying lengths. Aggressive voice therapy for 1 year is described if using this approach.[37]

Pulsed Dye Laser

Shown to be effective in the treatment of hypertrophic scars, Hwang and colleagues[30] studied the effect of pulsed dye laser treatment in 25 patients with sulcus vocalis. They showed improvement in pliability and vibration of the treated vocal fold as well as improvement in VHI scores.[30]

FUTURE INVESTIGATION

With the principal problem of sulcus vocalis a variable degeneration of the lamina propria, investigations over the past decade have focused on finding an ideal replacement material for lamina propria regeneration.[38] Within the field of tissue engineering, promising approaches to restoring a structurally compromised vocal fold are being investigated.[32,39] Studies examining the effect of hyaluronic acid and collagen-derived scaffolds on scarred vocal folds have been published.[40] Atelocollagen sheet implantation into the vocal fold lamina propria has shown the ability to regenerate the extracellular matrix with vocal fold fibroblast proliferation.[26]

In vivo animal experiments with molecular markers and cell therapy have shown great potential. Transforming growth factor β3 has been found to have a role in vocal fold repair mechanisms by modulating fibroblast differentiation and interrupting macrophage recruitment.[41] Other studies have shown that scar tissue fibroblasts cultured with adipose-derived stem cells produce less collagen and more antifibrotic properties.[42] Grafting small-intestinal submucosa into the vocal fold of a canine model resulted in newly generated hyaluronic acid and has the potential for treating vocal fold scar/sulcus.[43]

Hepatocyte growth factor (HGF), which is known to have therapeutic potential for other fibrotic diseases, also plays a promising role.[44] When locally injected into damaged canine vocal folds, HGF led to histologic regeneration and improved vibratory function.[45] Based on preclinical data and animal model studies, Hirano and colleagues in 2018[46] published their results of the first phase I/II clinical trial for intracordal injection of recombinant HGF for vocal fold scar and sulcus in 18 human patients. Their results are encouraging with no safety concerns noted, an improvement in patients' VHI-10 scores, and improvement in vocal fold vibratory function.[46] Given these promising outcomes, plans for a phase III, placebo-controlled clinical trial is in progress.

SUMMARY

The diagnosis and treatment of sulcus vocalis can be both challenging and rewarding. Voice therapy, endoscopic, and open treatment options should be considered and tailored to individual functional limitations and expectations. On the horizon are further investigations into tissue engineering, stem cell therapy, and novel restoration techniques to the human vocal fold architecture and molecular biomechanics.

REFERENCES

1. Hirano M. Morphological structure of the vocal cord as a vibrator and its variations. Folia Phoniatr (Basel) 1974;26(2):89–94.
2. Luchsinger R. Physiology of the voice. Folia Phoniatr (Basel) 1953;5(2):58–127 [in Undetermined Language].
3. Bouchayer M, Cornut G, Witzig E, et al. Epidermoid cysts, sulci, and mucosal bridges of the true vocal cord: a report of 157 cases. Laryngoscope 1985; 95(9 Pt 1):1087–94.
4. Itoh T, Kawasaki H, Morikawa I, et al. Vocal fold furrows. A 10-year review of 240 patients. Auris Nasus Larynx 1983;10(Suppl):S17–26.
5. Ford CN, Inagi K, Khidr A, et al. Sulcus vocalis: a rational analytical approach to diagnosis and management. Ann Otol Rhinol Laryngol 1996;105(3):189–200.
6. Giovanni A, Chanteret C, Lagier A. Sulcus vocalis: a review. Eur Arch Otorhinolaryngol 2007;264(4):337–44.
7. Selleck AM, Moore JE, Rutt AL, et al. Sulcus vocalis (type III): prevalence and strobovideolaryngoscopy characteristics. J Voice 2015;29(4):507–11.
8. Karle WE, Helman SN, Cooper A, et al. Temporalis fascia transplantation for sulcus vocalis and vocal fold scar: long-term outcomes. Ann Otol Rhinol Laryngol 2018;127(4):223–8.
9. Rosen CA. Vocal fold scar: evaluation and treatment. Otolaryngol Clin North Am 2000;33(5):1081–6.
10. Hirano M, Yoshida T, Tanaka S, et al. Sulcus vocalis: functional aspects. Ann Otol Rhinol Laryngol 1990;99(9 Pt 1):679–83.
11. Sato K, Hirano M. Electron microscopic investigation of sulcus vocalis. Ann Otol Rhinol Laryngol 1998;107(1):56–60.
12. Pinto JA, da Silva Freitas ML, Carpes AF, et al. Autologous grafts for treatment of vocal sulcus and atrophy. Otolaryngol Head Neck Surg 2007;137(5):785–91.
13. Nakayama M, Ford CN, Brandenburg JH, et al. Sulcus vocalis in laryngeal cancer: a histopathologic study. Laryngoscope 1994;104(1 Pt 1):16–24.
14. Monday LA, Cornut G, Bouchayer M, et al. Epidermoid cysts of the vocal cords. Ann Otol Rhinol Laryngol 1983;92(2 Pt 1):124–7.
15. Husain S, Sulica L. Familial sulcus vergeture: further evidence for congenital origin of type 2 sulcus. J Voice 2016;30(6). 761.e19-e21.
16. Lee A, Sulica L, Aylward A, et al. Sulcus vocalis: a new clinical paradigm based on a re-evaluation of histology. Laryngoscope 2016;126(6):1397–403.
17. Poels PJ, de Jong FI, Schutte HK. Consistency of the preoperative and intraoperative diagnosis of benign vocal fold lesions. J Voice 2003;17(3):425–33.

18. Dailey SH, Spanou K, Zeitels SM. The evaluation of benign glottic lesions: rigid telescopic stroboscopy versus suspension microlaryngoscopy. J Voice 2007; 21(1):112–8.

19. Akbulut S, Altintas H, Oguz H. Videolaryngostroboscopy versus microlaryngoscopy for the diagnosis of benign vocal cord lesions: a prospective clinical study. Eur Arch Otorhinolaryngol 2015;272(1):131–6.

20. Lindestad PA, Hertegard S. Spindle-shaped glottal insufficiency with and without sulcus vocalis: a retrospective study. Ann Otol Rhinol Laryngol 1994;103(7): 547–53.

21. Rajasudhakar R. Effect of voice therapy in sulcus vocalis: a single case study. S Afr J Commun Disord 2016;63(1):e1–5.

22. Miaskiewicz B, Szkielkowska A, Gos E, et al. Pathological sulcus vocalis: treatment approaches and voice outcomes in 36 patients. Eur Arch Otorhinolaryngol 2018;275(11):2763–71.

23. Ford CN. Advances and refinements in phonosurgery. Laryngoscope 1999; 109(12):1891–900.

24. Welham NV, Choi SH, Dailey SH, et al. Prospective multi-arm evaluation of surgical treatments for vocal fold scar and pathologic sulcus vocalis. Laryngoscope 2011;121(6):1252–60.

25. Sung CK, Tsao GJ. Single-operator flexible nasolaryngoscopy-guided transthyrohyoid vocal fold injections. Ann Otol Rhinol Laryngol 2013;122(1):9–14.

26. Kishimoto Y, Welham NV, Hirano S. Implantation of atelocollagen sheet for vocal fold scar. Curr Opin Otolaryngol Head Neck Surg 2010;18(6):507–11.

27. Ford CN, Bless DM. Selected problems treated by vocal fold injection of collagen. Am J Otolaryngol 1993;14(4):257–61.

28. Ford CN, Bless DM, Campbell D. Studies of injectable soluble collagen for vocal fold augmentation. Rev Laryngol Otol Rhinol (Bord) 1987;108(1):33–6.

29. Su CY, Tsai SS, Chiu JF, et al. Medialization laryngoplasty with strap muscle transposition for vocal fold atrophy with or without sulcus vocalis. Laryngoscope 2004; 114(6):1106–12.

30. Hwang CS, Lee HJ, Ha JG, et al. Use of pulsed dye laser in the treatment of sulcus vocalis. Otolaryngol Head Neck Surg 2013;148(5):804–9.

31. Remacle M, Lawson G, Degols JC, et al. Microsurgery of sulcus vergeture with carbon dioxide laser and injectable collagen. Ann Otol Rhinol Laryngol 2000; 109(2):141–8.

32. Ling C, Li Q, Brown ME, et al. Bioengineered vocal fold mucosa for voice restoration. Sci Transl Med 2015;7(314):314ra187.

33. Neuenschwander MC, Sataloff RT, Abaza MM, et al. Management of vocal fold scar with autologous fat implantation: perceptual results. J Voice 2001;15(2): 295–304.

34. Sataloff RT, Spiegel JR, Hawkshaw MJ. Vocal fold scar. Ear Nose Throat J 1997; 76(11):776.

35. Sataloff RT, Spiegel JR, Hawkshaw M, et al. Autologous fat implantation for vocal fold scar: a preliminary report. J Voice 1997;11(2):238–46.

36. Tsunoda K, Kondou K, Kaga K, et al. Autologous transplantation of fascia into the vocal fold: long-term result of type-1 transplantation and the future. Laryngoscope 2005;115(12 Pt 2 Suppl 108):1–10.

37. Pontes P, Behlau M. Treatment of sulcus vocalis: auditory perceptual and acoustical analysis of the slicing mucosa surgical technique. J Voice 1993;7(4):365–76.

38. Kanemaru S, Nakamura T, Omori K, et al. Regeneration of the vocal fold using autologous mesenchymal stem cells. Ann Otol Rhinol Laryngol 2003;112(11): 915–20.
39. Chhetri DK, Head C, Revazova E, et al. Lamina propria replacement therapy with cultured autologous fibroblasts for vocal fold scars. Otolaryngol Head Neck Surg 2004;131(6):864–70.
40. Chan RW, Gray SD, Titze IR. The importance of hyaluronic acid in vocal fold biomechanics. Otolaryngol Head Neck Surg 2001;124(6):607–14.
41. Chang Z, Kishimoto Y, Hasan A, et al. TGF-beta3 modulates the inflammatory environment and reduces scar formation following vocal fold mucosal injury in rats. Dis Model Mech 2014;7(1):83–91.
42. Mattei A, Magalon J, Bertrand B, et al. Cell therapy and vocal fold scarring. Eur Ann Otorhinolaryngol Head Neck Dis 2017;134(5):339–45.
43. Pitman MJ, Cabin JA, Iacob CE. Small intestinal submucosa implantation for the possible treatment of vocal fold scar, sulcus, and superficial lamina propria atrophy. Ann Otol Rhinol Laryngol 2016;125(2):137–44.
44. Ohno T, Hirano S, Rousseau B. Gene expression of transforming growth factor-beta1 and hepatocyte growth factor during wound healing of injured rat vocal fold. Laryngoscope 2009;119(4):806–10.
45. Hirano S, Bless D, Heisey D, et al. Roles of hepatocyte growth factor and transforming growth factor beta1 in production of extracellular matrix by canine vocal fold fibroblasts. Laryngoscope 2003;113(1):144–8.
46. Hirano S, Kawamoto A, Tateya I, et al. A phase I/II exploratory clinical trial for intracordal injection of recombinant hepatocyte growth factor for vocal fold scar and sulcus. J Tissue Eng Regen Med 2018;12(4):1031–8.

Updated Medical and Surgical Treatment for Common Benign Laryngeal Lesions

Kristen L. Kraimer, BS[a], Inna Husain, MD[b],*

KEYWORDS

- Vocal fold polyp • Vocal fold cyst • Vocal process granuloma • Vocal fold nodules
- pKTP laser • Intralesional injection

KEY POINTS

- Controversy exists regarding nomenclature of benign vocal fold lesions but advancements in visualization, stroboscopy, and response to therapy aid in describing specific lesions.
- Vocal fold nodules are typically responsive to voice therapy, and intralesional steroid injection, both in the operating room and office settings, can aid in resolution of these lesions.
- Vocal fold polyp management is similar to that of vocal fold nodules but angiolytic laser treatment has recently been studied as another effective treatment modality.
- Vocal fold cyst treatment traditionally differs from that of nodules or polyps but recent studies using intralesional injections and angiolytic laser therapy demonstrate efficacy.
- Vocal process granuloma treatment has expanded from management of risk factors to now include use of botulinum toxin injection and angiolytic laser therapy.

 Video content accompanies this article at http://www.oto.theclinics.com.

INTRODUCTION

Benign laryngeal lesions are often the result of phonotraumatic forces on the vocal folds and thus classically are treated with a combination of voice therapy and phonomicrosurgical techniques to minimize inadvertent additional trauma. Despite growing

Disclosure Statement: The authors have no commercial or financial conflicts of interest to report.
[a] Rush Medical College, 600 S. Paulina Street, Suite 202, Chicago, IL 60612, USA; [b] Rush University Medical Center, 1611 West Harrison, Suite 550, Chicago, IL 60612, USA
* Corresponding author.
E-mail address: Inna_husain@rush.edu

Otolaryngol Clin N Am 52 (2019) 745–757
https://doi.org/10.1016/j.otc.2019.03.017
0030-6665/19/© 2019 Elsevier Inc. All rights reserved.

oto.theclinics.com

literature on treatment modality for these lesions, controversy regarding appropriate nomenclature remains, which leads to confusion among providers and researchers for benign laryngeal lesions. Rosen and colleagues[1] developed a nomenclature paradigm to address this issue that involved analysis of stroboscopy, response to voice therapy, and surgical findings to classify these lesions. Analyses such as these are useful to create common languages among laryngologists and otolaryngologists treating benign laryngeal lesions. Although controversy and ambiguity exist in nomenclature, treatment modalities for these lesions are often quite similar.

Many benign vocal fold lesions arise from some component of phonotrauma. Vocal misuse or overuse results in midmembranous mechanical stress leading to wound healing and remodeling. The trauma and healing process give rise to a variety of lesions that can be further classified by appearance and stroboscopy, although differentiating some lesions may be unclear. Because of the role of phonotrauma in the development of vocal fold lesions, voice therapy is a key component of treatment plans that address, heal, and prevent future lesions.

VOCAL FOLD NODULES
Cause

Vocal fold nodules are a common laryngeal pathologic condition that are typically caused by vocal misuse or overuse and are demonstrated in **Figs. 1** and **2**. Over time, these voice behaviors lead to mechanical stress on the vocal folds and the development of nodules. Marcotullio and colleagues[2] found that vocal fold nodules tend to be associated with earlier changes in the lamina propria than lesions such as polyps. This suggests that nodules may indicate more recent manifestation of phonotrauma than polyps, 2 closely related benign lesions.

Management

Voice therapy
Voice therapy continues to be the mainstay of treatment for vocal fold nodules and may often be combined with other treatment modalities for recurrent or intractable nodules. Voice therapy typically consists of behavioral and habit modification, vocal hygiene education, increasing hydration, and avoidance of throat clearing.

Surgery
Phonomicrosurgery has been shown to be an effective treatment modality for vocal fold nodules. A study by Uloza and colleagues[3] demonstrated significantly improved

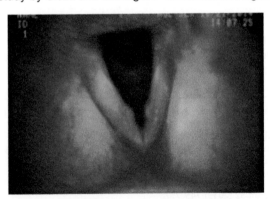

Fig. 1. Transnasal distal chip laryngoscopy demonstrating bilateral vocal fold nodules in a waitress.

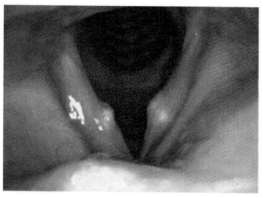

Fig. 2. Transnasal distal chip laryngoscopy demonstrating bilateral vocal fold nodules, left greater than right, with overlying keratosis. Subject is a daycare teacher.

visual analog scores and significantly decreased grade, rough, and breathy scores in patients treated with phonomicrosurgery versus controls. There have been several recent studies highlighting strategies to augment the benefits of surgical excision. Voice therapy following surgery has been shown to decrease the recurrence rate of nodules as shown in a retrospective study of 62 patients in which absence of postoperative voice therapy was associated with a significantly higher nodule recurrence rate.[4]

Intralesional injection
Newer management options, including intralesional steroid injections, have been shown to improve resolution of these nodules. In a retrospective cohort study of 211 patients with vocal polyps, nodules, or cysts, patients who underwent intralesional triamcinolone injections at the time of laryngeal microsurgery were compared against those who underwent laryngeal microsurgery alone. In the group with intralesional steroid injection there was a significantly lower rate of recurrence and risk of persistent dysphonia.[5] This is thought to be due to reduction in scar formation and granulation tissue formation from the surgical excision. In a retrospective case series, Wang and colleagues[6] demonstrated improved nodule regression rate with transoral injection of triamcinolone and dexamethasone as compared with voice hygiene education alone. Mortenson and Woo discussed the use of office laryngeal steroid injection to reduce granulation tissue to promote primary healing, reduce hypertrophic scar formation, and to reduce inflammation to avoid surgical intervention in patients with vocal fold nodules, polyps, scars, and granulomas.[7] In addition, intralesional steroid injections can be done serially in the office, providing treatment for the patient without the cost, time, and morbidity of several operating room treatment sessions. Photographic examples of this procedure are shown in **Figs. 3** and **4** depicting transcervical and transnasal approaches, respectively. This can be an awake intervention as well, allowing the patient to avoid anesthetic risks and time spent for the entire procedure.

VOCAL FOLD POLYPS
Cause

Vocal fold polyps represent another common benign vocal fold lesion. As described by Marcotullio and colleagues,[2] a vocal fold polyp is an abnormal, unilateral growth of a vocal fold and typically consists of later stages of lamina propria wound healing

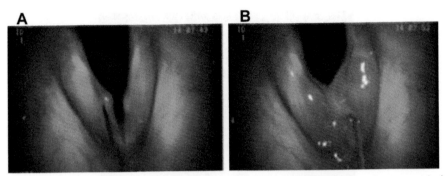

Fig. 3. In-office awake intralesional steroid injections of vocal fold nodules, via transcervical route through the thyrohyoid membrane. (*A*) Vocal fold nodules before injection. (*B*) Vocal fold nodules after intralesional steroid injection.

after phonotrauma as compared with vocal fold nodules. Recent studies have further characterized polyps to understand the pathophysiology of these lesions. Gene expression in extracellular matrix proteins has been studied to characterize these lesions. A study by Thibeault and colleagues[8] demonstrated that vocal fold polyps had upregulation of procollagen and increased expression of fibronectin, which can lead to severe mucosal wave stiffness and inflammatory gene association. The study also demonstrated the presence of hyaluronic acid synthase 2 and hyaluronidase messenger RNA, indicating active turnover and remodeling in the polyp sample.[8] In addition, a study by Wang and colleagues[9] demonstrated a significantly higher expression of pepsin in patients with vocal fold polyps as compared with the study controls. This suggests a potential role for laryngopharyngeal reflux in the development of the vocal fold polyps.

Management Options

Management of vocal fold polyps is more controversial than that of vocal fold nodules and includes voice therapy, surgical excision, intralesional steroid injection, and angiolytic laser treatment although surgical excision continues to be the mainstay treatment option. **Fig. 5** demonstrates an example of phonomicrosurgical excision of vocal fold polyps.

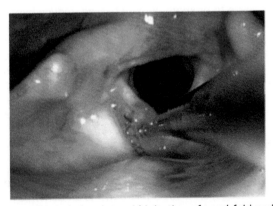

Fig. 4. Flexible transnasal intralesional steroid injection of vocal fold nodules.

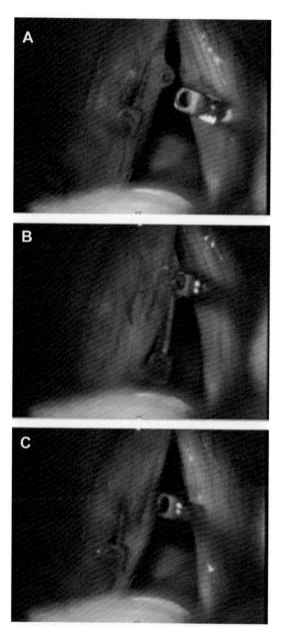

Fig. 5. Phonomicrosurgical technique for resection of left vocal fold polyp. (*A*) Polyp is visualized along the anterior medial border of the left vocal fold. (*B*) Polyp is retracted medially and truncated at the base with laryngeal microscissors. (*C*) Postexcision appearance of left vocal fold.

Voice therapy

Although surgical intervention is the standard intervention, there may also be a role for voice therapy in the treatment of vocal fold polyps. A large retrospective study of 644 patients compared conservative treatment with voice therapy or medication to surgical treatment with excision.[10] Of this population, 9.7% of patients had complete resolution with conservative treatment, indicating that some patients may improve without the typical surgical intervention.[10] A randomized controlled trial of 150 patients studied exclusive voice therapy as a treatment for polyps using "voice expulsion therapy."[11] This consisted of 2 stages of voice therapy treatment, with the first stage focusing on exercises to induce laryngeal microtrauma followed by another stage of typical voice therapy. The study compared microsurgery plus voice therapy or voice expulsion therapy and found no significant difference between the groups clinically or in patients' subjective satisfaction.[11] Although "voice expulsion therapy" is not a common practice, this study demonstrates a potential role of sole voice therapy in treatment of polyp. Future study to elucidate patient characteristics that can make patients more likely to respond to voice therapy or surgery is important.

Intralesional injections
Like treatment for vocal fold nodules, intralesional steroid injections have been studied for treating vocal fold polyps. Similar to treatment for vocal fold nodules, intralesional steroid injections can be performed with the patient awake in the office, decreasing time and cost for the patient to receive effective treatment for their polyps. A study by Wang and colleagues[6] demonstrated improvement with steroid injections but noted common recurrence of symptoms and lesions. Hsu and colleagues[12] demonstrated a 91% response rate to percutaneous steroid injection and a complete remission rate of 59%. Despite a significant improvement between preoperative and postoperative GRBAS scores, 41% of patients did not experience complete remission, indicating need for further study in patient characteristics to understand which patients may be appropriate for treatment solely with steroid injection.[12] Steroid injections immediately following surgical excision have also been studied. A retrospective cohort study of patients with vocal polyps, nodules, and cyst demonstrated a 0.3-fold decrease in the odds ratio in the risk of persistent dysphonia and a significantly lower rate of recurrence in patients treated with adjunctive steroid injection during laryngeal microsurgery as compared with those who underwent laryngeal microsurgery excision alone.[5]

Laser treatment
Laser treatment of vocal fold polyps has also been recently studied as an alternative to cold excision. In a study comparing angiolytic laser surgery with microflap excision, both methods demonstrated significant improvements in symptomology and no significant differences between the treatment methods in regard to aerodynamic or acoustic functions.[13] This demonstrates the utility of angiolytic laser surgery as an alternative to the more traditional microflap excision. Potassium-titanyl-phosphate (KTP) laser is a photoangiolytic laser that operates at a wavelength of 532 nm, similar to the absorption spectrum of oxyhemoglobin, to specifically target damage to red blood cells and microvasculature while avoiding injury to surrounding epithelium and superficial lamina propria of the vocal folds. Using this laser on pulsed versus continuous mode has been discussed as a method to avoid ablating extravascular tissue.[14] The KTP laser has been used to treat benign laryngeal lesions and is used in the office clinic setting, as well as in the operating room. A multiinstitutional retrospective study evaluated 102 patients who underwent in-office KTP laser treatment of benign vocal fold lesions and found a significant reduction in lesion size.[15] The investigators found a significant reduction in lesion size at the first follow-up appointment in patient with granuloma, hemorrhagic polyp, leukoplakia, nonhemorrhagic polyp, and Reinke edema with significant reduction in long-term follow-up in patients with hemorrhagic

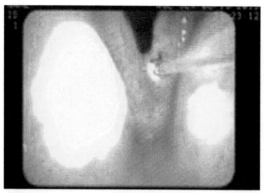

Fig. 6. Awake pKTP laser treatment of left vocal fold lesion.

polyp, leukoplakia, and nonhemorrhagic polyp.[15] **Fig. 6** and Video 1 demonstrate examples of pulsed KTP (pKTP) use.

pKTP excision has also been studied as an office-based approach to treatment of vocal fold polyps. A retrospective study by Sridharan and colleagues[16] demonstrated the utility of pKTP ablation of vocal fold polyps, with associated decrease in mean VHI-10 scores in all patients. Wang and colleagues[17] studied combining pKTP laser treatment with blunt removal via flexible laryngoscopy, to treatment with pKTP laser alone. In this approach, a 0.4-mm pKTP laser fiber is passed through the working channel of a flexible laryngoscope and used to coagulate the vocal fold polyp, which is then bluntly removed with flexible forceps via the same channel. They found significant improvement in maximal phonation time and VHI in the combination group 2 weeks postoperatively. Six weeks postoperatively, however, there was significant improvement in these measures in both groups, indicating that the removal of the cauterized tissue may confer an early therapeutic effect.[17] Another study compared the same procedure of pKTP polyp cauterization with blunt transnasal removal to excision of polyp via microlaryngeal surgery and found no significant differences in clinical improvement between the 2 groups.[18]

VOCAL FOLD CYSTS
Cause

Vocal fold cysts are typically classified as epidermal or mucous retention cysts and are thought to be due to vocal misuse, gastroesophageal reflux, or upper airway infection.[19] An image of a vocal fold cyst is included in **Fig. 7**. Epidermal cysts are thought to be caused by vocal abuse or epithelium confined within the lamina propria, whereas mucous retention cysts are due to gland obstruction.[19] Epidermal and mucous cysts are also differentiated by histology; the squamous inclusion cysts are covered with stratified squamous epithelium and mucous retention cysts are covered with ciliated epithelium.[19,20]

Vocal fold cysts can also be challenging to distinguish from pseudocysts, vocal sulci, and mucosal bridge lesions. Hernando and colleagues[21] discussed stroboscopy as an essential tool to use, in association with surgical findings, to differentiate and correctly diagnose these lesions. In addition, vocal fold cysts can present similarly to vocal fold polyps or nodules, so careful examination is essential for diagnosis.

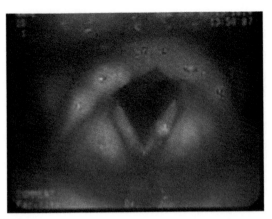

Fig. 7. Left vocal fold cyst.

Management

Surgical excision

Treatment options typically include surgical excision and voice therapy. Surgical excision with microflap excision of the lesion is recommended, as the lesions do not typically improve with conservative measures alone. An image during this procedure is shown in **Fig. 8**. A recent study by Tibbetts and colleagues[22] analyzed the role of perioperative voice therapy and found no significant benefit. Patients who underwent surgery with or without perioperative voice therapy both experienced significant improvement in their VHI-10 scores but there was no significant difference between the groups.[22] Despite this finding, there may be a role for voice therapy in postoperative wound healing after cyst excision that needs to be further studied.

Intralesional injection

Intralesional steroid injections have been used for treatment of these lesions. As discussed earlier, steroid injections have also been shown as an adequate treatment for vocal fold cysts.[6] In the study time of 24 months, symptom recurrence, VHI-10 scores, and need for further interventions were followed. The investigators found a 43% success rate, indicating that steroid injection may be a poor choice for some patients and should be considered when counseling patients in treatment options.[6] Steroid

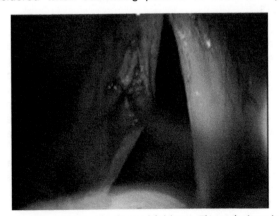

Fig. 8. Phonomicrosurgical excision of left vocal fold cyst. The technique involves creating a microflap for submucosal resection.

injections have also been studied as an adjunct to surgical excision and are associated with a significant decrease in persistent dysphonia when compared with microlaryngeal surgery alone[5]; this demonstrates the utility of adjunctive steroid injection to treat vocal folds cysts.

Laser excision

Carbon dioxide (CO_2) laser microsurgery has been used to treat vocal fold cysts. A retrospective review of 49 patients treated with excision via microflap created with CO_2 laser demonstrated significant improvements in grade of dysphonia, VHI, and maximum phonation time.[23] This exhibited the efficacy of the newer AcuBlade CO_2 laser system for treatment without major thermal damage to surrounding epithelium or lamina propria. The study demonstrated the utility of laser treatment and provided an alternative surgical technique to classic cold phonomicrosurgery. A recent report by Izadi and colleagues[24] describes an island flap technique for intracordal mucous retention cyst using a CO_2 laser for lesion excision. In this small prospective study of 4 patients, the investigators found this to be an effective treatment modality but in need of comparison with other treatments.

pKTP laser treatment has been studied to treat vocal fold cysts (and a variety of other benign vocal fold lesions) in a study by Sheu and colleagues. The investigators were able to show that all lesions reduced in size.[16] This study only included 2 cases of vocal fold cyst and only one that continued in follow-up analysis, so additional larger studies are needed to draw broader conclusions specifically for vocal fold cysts. Another study analyzed laryngeal lesion size reduction with in-office pKTP treatment and found a reduction in size for vocal fold cysts, although only one patient with this lesion was included in the cohort.[25] Further study for the specific use of pKTP laser in vocal fold cysts will be useful to better understand treatment parameters and expectations for lesion improvement.

VOCAL PROCESS GRANULOMA
Cause

Vocal process granuloma (VPG) is a benign laryngeal lesion typically caused by trauma secondary to intubation, voice misuse, or gastroesophageal reflux disease. These lesions were first described by Chevalier Jackson in 1928 as "contact ulcers" and have had several names over time and as the known causes have expanded.[26] Most of these lesions are located at the vocal process of the arytenoid and may be caused by iatrogenic trauma, behavioral trauma, or chronic irritation.[27] Voice misuse, especially repetitive throat clearing or coughing, has been described as a cause for the development of this lesion due to the pressure that forceful glottic closure creates.[28] An image of a vocal process granuloma is shown in **Fig. 9**. In an early study by Öhman and colleagues,[29] esophageal dysfunction, as measured by pH monitoring, acid perfusion test, and acid clearing tests, was present in 74% of the patients studied in one cohort study of vocal contact ulcers, as compared with a rate of 30% esophageal dysfunction in the general population. Treatment of these lesions can be challenging due to multifactorial cause and high recurrence rates. Recurrence rates for VPGs have been shown to be as high as 90% and have led to challenging decision-making for treatment and several tiers of treatment modalities.[30]

Management

Antireflux medical therapy

A systematic review by Karkos and colleagues[30] discussed treatment recommendations for these lesions. Conservative treatment of vocal process granuloma includes

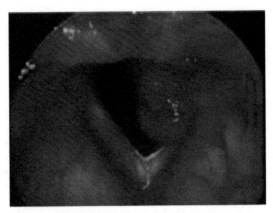

Fig. 9. Large left vocal process granuloma.

antireflux therapy with proton pump inhibitors, speech and language therapy, and inhaled steroids. Leonard and Kendall retrospectively studied the utility of antireflux medication with voice therapy to treat VPGs and found no recurrences among the 8 patients who completed the voice therapy program in the 1 to 2 years of study follow-up.[31] This emphasized the likely multifactorial component of vocal process granuloma development and utility of treatment with several modalities.

Botulinum toxin injection

Refractory lesions have been treated with botulinum toxin injection, with several studies demonstrating resolution rates of 100%.[30] **Fig. 10** depicts an image of this procedure. Fink and colleagues[32] described injection into the interarytenoid muscle in the office of 8 patients who had failed surgical, medical, or voice therapy, with 5 patients demonstrating complete resolution. In patients with vocal process granulomas and glottic insufficiency, autologous fat injection laryngoplasty has been studied as a treatment.[33] Improving glottic closure in this manner is thought to decrease laryngeal hyperfunction, thus improving the vocal process granuloma, and this was seen in 7 of the 9 patients in the study with complete resolution and partial resolution in the remaining patients.[33] A recent prospective cohort study by Lei and colleagues[34]

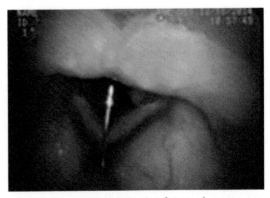

Fig. 10. Intraarytenoid botulinum toxin A injection for vocal process granuloma (on left) via transcervical approach through the thyrohyoid membrane.

compared treatment with antireflux medications, esomeprazole plus mosapride citrate (a promotility drug), versus botulinum toxin injection and found a significant improvement in symptoms in the antireflux medication group. Further large, randomized studies are needed to understand a potential treatment advantage further to develop stronger evidence-based treatment guidelines.

Surgical and laser excision

Surgical management has included cold microlaryngeal surgery, carbon dioxide laser treatment, and pKTP laser treatment. Karkos and colleagues[30] describe indications for surgical intervention as failure of medical management, airway obstruction, and biopsy if malignancy is suspected. A recent study by Dominguez and colleagues[35] retrospectively studied pKTP laser ablation of vocal fold granulomas in 26 patients and noted complete resolution in 73.1% of cases with no recurrence in these patients, which demonstrates the possibility of in-office treatment with pKTP laser for these lesions.

SUMMARY

Benign vocal fold lesions encompass several distinct lesions, each with specific diagnostic and treatment modalities. However, nomenclature discrepancies exist in the literature and lead to confusion when studying and treating these lesions. Voice therapy is a key component of treatment for most lesions because phonotrauma is usually involved in the pathogenesis of these lesions. Newer treatment modalities include awake, outpatient procedures such as intralesional steroid injection and pKTP laser treatment. These can often be used as an adjunct to more traditional phonomicrosurgical techniques, both in the operating room and in the office. Voice therapy techniques also continue to evolve and, as diagnostic differences among lesions improve, some voice therapy modalities may be recommended based on lesion type. As office-based procedure technology continues to improve, patients will have access to more options for definitive treatment.

SUPPLEMENTARY DATA

Supplementary data related to this article can be found online at https://doi.org/10.1016/j.otc.2019.03.017.

REFERENCES

1. Rosen CA, Gartner-Schmidt J, Hathaway B, et al. A nomenclature paradigm for benign midmembranous vocal fold lesions. Laryngoscope 2012;122:1335–41.
2. Marcotullio D, Magliulo G, Pietrunti S, et al. Exudative laryngeal diseases of Reinke's space: a clinicohistopathological framing. J Otolaryngol 2002;31:376–80.
3. Uloza V, Saferis V, Uloziene I. Perceptual and acoustic assessment of voice pathology and the efficacy of endolaryngeal phonomicrosurgery. J Voice 2005;19: 138–45.
4. Béquignon E, Bach C, Fugain C, et al. Long-term results of surgical treatment of vocal fold nodules. Laryngoscope 2013;123:1926–30.
5. Cho JH, Kim SY, Joo YH, et al. Efficacy and safety of adjunctive steroid injection after microsurgical removal of benign vocal fold lesions. J Voice 2017;31:615–20.
6. Wang CT, Lai MS, Cheng PW. Long-term surveillance following intralesional steroid injection for benign vocal fold lesions. JAMA Otolaryngol Head Neck Surg 2017;143:589–94.

7. Mortensen M, Woo P. Office steroid injections of the larynx. Laryngoscope 2006; 116:1735–9.

8. Thibeault SL, Gray S, Li W, et al. Genotypic and phenotypic expression of vocal fold polyps and Reinke's edema: a preliminary study. Ann Otol Rhinol Laryngol 2002;111:302–9.

9. Wang L, Tan JJ, Wu T, et al. Association between laryngeal pepsin levels and the presence of vocal fold polyps. Otolaryngol Head Neck Surg 2017;156:144–51.

10. Nakagawa H, Miyamoto M, Kusuyama T, et al. Resolution of vocal fold polyps with conservative treatment. J Voice 2012;26:e107–10.

11. Barillari MR, Volpe U, Mirra G, et al. Surgery or rehabilitation: a randomized clinical trial comparing the treatment of vocal fold polyps via phonosurgery and traditional voice therapy with "voice therapy expulsion" training. J Voice 2017;31: 379.e13–20.

12. Hsu YB, Lan MC, Chang SY. Percutaneous corticosteroid injection for vocal fold polyp. Arch Otolaryngol Head Neck Surg 2009;135:776–80.

13. Mizuta M, Hiwatashi N, Kobayashi T, et al. Comparison of vocal outcomes after angiolytic laser surgery and microflap surgery for vocal polyps. Auris Nasus Larynx 2015;42:453–7.

14. Zeitels SM, Burns JA. Office-based laryngeal laser surgery with the 532-nm pulsed-potassium-titanyl-phosphate laser. Curr Opin Otolaryngol Head Neck Surg 2007;15:394–400.

15. Sheu M, Sridharan S, Kuhn M, et al. Multi-institutional experience with the in-office potassium titanyl phosphate laser for laryngeal lesions. J Voice 2012;26:806–10.

16. Sridharan S, Achlatis S, Ruiz R, et al. Patient-based outcomes of in-office KTP ablation of vocal fold polyps. Laryngoscope 2014;124:1176–9.

17. Wang CT, Huang TW, Liao LJ, et al. Office-based potassium titanyl phosphate laser-assisted endoscopic vocal polypectomy. JAMA Otolaryngol Head Neck Surg 2013;139:610–6.

18. Wang CT, Liao LJ, Huang TW, et al. Comparison of treatment outcomes of transnasal vocal fold polypectomy versus microlaryngoscopic surgery. Laryngoscope 2015;125:1155–60.

19. Martins RH, Santana MF, Tavares EL. Vocal cysts: clinical, endoscopic, and surgical aspects. J Voice 2011;25:107–10.

20. Johns MM. Update on the etiology, diagnosis, and treatment of vocal fold nodules, polyps, and cysts. Curr Opin Otolaryngol Head Neck Surg 2003;11:456–61.

21. Hernando M, Cobeta I, Lara A, et al. Vocal pathologies of difficult diagnosis. J Voice 2008;22:607–10.

22. Tibbetts KM, Dominguez LM, Simpson CB. Impact of perioperative voice therapy on outcomes in the surgical management of vocal fold cysts. J Voice 2018;32: 347–51.

23. Matar N, Amoussa K, Verduyckt I, et al. CO2 laser-assisted microsurgery for intracordal cysts: technique and results of 49 patients. Eur Arch Otorhinolaryngol 2010;267:1905–9.

24. Izadi F, Ghanbari H, Zahedi S, et al. An island flap technique for laryngeal intracordal mucous retention cysts. Iran J Otorhinolaryngol 2015;27:337–42.

25. Mallur PS, Tajudeen BA, Aaronson N, et al. Quantification of benign lesion regression as a function of 532-nm pulsed potassium titanyl phosphate laser parameter selection. Laryngoscope 2011;121:590–5.

26. Jackson C. Contact ulcer of the larynx. Ann Otol Rhinol Laryngol 1928;37:228–30.

27. Bradley PJ. Arytenoid granuloma. J Laryngol Otol 1997;111:801–3.

28. Devaney KO, Rinaldo A, Ferlito A. Vocal process granuloma of the larynx—recognition, differential diagnosis and treatment. Oral Oncol 2005;41:666–9.
29. Öhman L, Tibbling L, Olofsson J, et al. Esophageal dysfunction in patients with contact ulcer of the larynx. Ann Otol Rhinol Laryngol 1928;92:228–30.
30. Karkos PD, George M, Van Der Veen J, et al. Vocal process granulomas: a systematic review of treatment. Ann Otol Rhinol Laryngol 2014;123:314–20.
31. Leonard R, Kendall K. Effects of voice therapy on vocal process granuloma: a phonoscopic approach. Am J Otolaryngol 2005;26:101–7.
32. Fink DS, Achkar J, Franco RA, et al. Interarytenoid botulinum toxin injection for recalcitrant vocal process granuloma. Laryngoscope 2013;123:3084–7.
33. Hu HC, Hung YT, Lin SY, et al. Office-based autologous fat injection laryngoplasty for vocal process granuloma. J Voice 2016;30:758.e7–11.
34. Lei L, Yang H, Zhang X, et al. Comparison of the effects of esomeprazole plus mosapride citrate and botulinum toxin A on vocal process granuloma. Am J Otolaryngol 2017;38:593–7.
35. Dominguez LM, Brown RJ, Simpson CB. Treatment outcomes of in-office KTP ablation of vocal fold granulomas. Ann Otol Rhinol Laryngol 2017;126:829–34.

Movement Disorders and Voice

Grace Snow, MD[a], Elizabeth Guardiani, MD[b],*

KEYWORDS

- Laryngeal dystonia • Spasmodic dysphonia • Movement disorders
- Parkinson disease • Essential voice tremor • Botulinum toxin

KEY POINTS

- The diagnosis of movement disorders affecting the voice should be made based on history and clinical findings.
- Spasmodic dysphonia is a focal laryngeal dystonia where involuntary task-specific contractions of the laryngeal musculature affect the fluency of speech.
- Essential voice tremor may occur as a manifestation of essential tremor or isolated to the voice, causing periodic, oscillatory movements of the larynx and the resonance tract.
- Botulinum toxin injections to affected muscles of the larynx are an effective treatment in both spasmodic dysphonia and essential voice tremor.
- Parkinson disease is characterized by bradykinesia plus rest tremor and/or rigidity, and vocal complaints are treated most commonly with Lee Silverman Voice Treatment.

INTRODUCTION

Movement disorders are neurologic syndromes in which increased or decreased voluntary and involuntary movements occur that are unrelated to weakness or spasticity.[1] Movement disorders affecting the voice can impair patients' quality of life significantly. Movement disorders of the larynx may be isolated to the larynx as in spasmodic dysphonia (SD) or they may be part of a systemic neurologic process. Hyperfunctional movement disorders include dystonia and essential tremor (ET). Parkinson disease (PD) is a hypofunctional movement disorder. Myasthenia gravis and amyotrophic lateral sclerosis are also neurologic diseases that can affect the voice but are not categorized as movement disorders. Cerebrovascular accidents also can cause significant alternations in speech and laryngeal function. Patients with movement disorders affecting the voice may be referred to otolaryngologists

Disclosure Statement: The authors have nothing to disclose.
[a] Otorhinolaryngology Head and Neck Surgery, University of Maryland School of Medicine, 16 South Eutaw Street, Suite 500, Baltimore, MD 21201, USA; [b] University of Maryland School of Medicine, 16 South Eutaw Street, Suite 500, Baltimore, MD 21201, USA
* Corresponding author.
E-mail address: eguardiani@som.umaryland.edu

Otolaryngol Clin N Am 52 (2019) 759–767
https://doi.org/10.1016/j.otc.2019.03.018
0030-6665/19/Published by Elsevier Inc.
oto.theclinics.com

for treatment or may initially present to an otolaryngologist with voice complaints related to an undiagnosed movement disorder. Accurate diagnosis of a movement disorder allows appropriate management of the patient.

LARYNGEAL DYSTONIA/SPASMODIC DYSPHONIA

Laryngeal dystonia (LD) is characterized by task-specific involuntary contractions of laryngeal musculature. Most LDs are focal in that they affect only the larynx, but LD also can occur as part of segmental or generalized dystonia. SD is the most common form of LD and the terms are often used interchangeably. SD is a focal dystonia that affects the fluency of speech.[2] The exact pathophysiology of SD remains unknown, but it is generally believed a disorder of the central nervous system. Loss of cortical inhibition, sensory input disturbances, and neuroanatomic changes all seem implicated.[3] Although most cases of SD occur spontaneously, approximately 12% of patients have a family history of dystonia.[4]

Phenomenology

The most common form of SD is adductor SD (AdSD), which comprises approximately 80% to 90% of cases of SD.[2,5] It is characterized by a strained and strangled voice quality as well as voice breaks with abrupt initiation and termination of sound. Abductor SD (AbSD) comprises most of the remaining cases of LD and is characterized by breathy breaks during speech. Rarer forms of LD include mixed AbSD/AdSD, where patients have features of both AdSD and AbSD; singer's LD, where patients only have symptoms during singing; and adductor breathing LD, where adductor spasms occur during breathing resulting in stridor[4,6]; 25% of patients with SD have an accompanying irregular dystonic tremor of the larynx with phonation.[2] As with many patients with dystonia, patients with SD may be able to use a sensory trick, such as touching their face or speaking in an accent or an altered pitch, to temporarily improve the voice.[2] Symptoms also may be less pronounced with shouting, whispering, singing, laughing, and crying, but in contrast to muscle tension dysphonia, patients with SD typically do not report periods of entirely normal speech.[7,8] Approximately half of patients with LD have improvement in their symptoms with alcohol intake.[9]

Diagnosis

LD is diagnosed clinically, based primarily on history, voice, and laryngoscopic findings. Patients are asked to read sentences with repeating voiced vowels, commonly referred to as adductor sentences, as well as sentences with repeating voiceless consonants, commonly referred to as abductor sentences, and observed for the presence of voice breaks (**Table 1**).[8] Patients with AdSD have more breaks on the adductor sentences and patients with AbSD have more breaks on the abductor sentences; if a

Table 1 Sentences for eliciting voice breaks/laryngeal spasms in spasmodic dysphonia	
Adductor Sentences	**Abductor Sentences**
"Tom wants to be in the army."	"He is hiding behind the house."
"We eat eels every Easter."	"Patty helped Kathy carve the turkey."
"He was angry about it all year."	"Harry is happy because he has a new horse."
"He hurt his arm on the iron bar."	"During babyhood he had only half a head of hair"
"We mow our lawn all year."	"Who says a mahogany highboy isn't heavy?"

patient has equal difficulty with both groups of sentences, this is more likely to represent muscle tension dysphonia or less likely a true mixed LD. Flexible nasolaryngoscopy/stroboscopy is preferred over rigid stroboscopy because it allows for more physiologic voice production. The patient is asked to perform several vocal tasks, including prolonged vowel sounds, counting, and abductor and adductor sentences. The larynx is assessed for any anatomic etiology of dysphonia, the presence or absence of tremor, and any adductor or abductor spasms. There are no standard diagnostic criteria for SD, and a recent multicenter observational study demonstrated poor interrater agreement after viewing speech and nasolaryngoscopy video recordings.[10] Other tools, such as laryngeal electromyography, acoustic and aerodynamic analysis, and high-speed laryngoscopy, also have been used, particularly to measure response to treatment, but none offers any diagnostic certainty.[7]

Treatment

Botulinum toxin injections to the affected laryngeal musculature remains the standard treatment of LD/SD.[11] Injections typically are performed transcutaneously with electromyographic guidance. In AdSD, bilateral injection of the thyroarytenoid muscles is the most common technique, usually at a starting dose of 1 U each.[4] In AbSD, injection of the posterior cricoarytenoid muscle is performed in a staged fashion to avoid narrowing of the airway, usually at starting dose of 3.75 U.[4] The cricothyroid muscles also are occasionally treated in the treatment of AbSD as are the interarytenoid muscles in the treatment of AdSD.[12] Dosages vary widely among patients, and trial and error to find the best dosing regimen for each patient is required. Once a dosing regimen is established, however, it tends to stay stable over time.[13] Oral medications are not commonly used for SD; however, drugs like clonazepam, trihexyphenidyl, and baclofen sometimes are used as adjunct treatment to botulinum toxin injections, particularly in AbSD.[4] Sodium oxybate is an oral medication with a therapeutic effect similar to alcohol, which was shown to reduce voice symptoms in patients with alcohol-responsive SD.[14] Voice therapy is generally believed not an effective treatment of SD; however, it can be useful when the alternate diagnosis of muscle tension dysphonia is considered.

Surgical treatment of SD also may be considered as an alternative to botulinum toxin injections. Medialization laryngoplasty has been shown safe and effective in the treatment of AbSD.[15] The selective laryngeal adductor denervation-reinnervation procedure (**Fig. 1**) has been used to treat patients with AdSD successfully, with durable results in most patients.[16,17] Other less commonly performed procedures include myomectomy of affected laryngeal muscles and type II thyroplasty. In a small series of patients with AdSD, electrical stimulation of the thyroarytenoid muscles via an implanted device showed an improvement in voice, which may indicate a future direction for treatment.[18]

ESSENTIAL VOICE TREMOR

Essential voice tremor (EVT) is the manifestation of ET in the phonatory apparatus.[19] ET is defined as a mixed kinetic (occurring with movement) and postural tremor, which is not task specific and occurs in the absence of other neurologic symptoms. EVT affects approximately 10% to 25% of patients with ET[20] and results in a tremulous voice that persists across all vocal tasks.[19] EVT also can occur as the sole or predominant manifestation of ET and is referred to as isolated vocal tremor.[20] Approximately one-third to one-half have a family history of tremor, and 26% to 62% have some improvement in their voice with alcohol.[19–21]

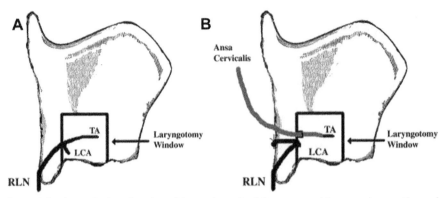

Fig. 1. (*A*) Schematic showing the adductor branch of the recurrent laryngeal nerve through a window created in the thyroid cartilage. (*B*) Schematic showing the cut proximal edge of the adductor branch and the ansa cervicalis anastomosed to the distal branch. LCA, lateral cricoarytenoid muscle; RLN, Recurrent laryngeal nerve; TA, thyroarytenoid muscle. (*From* Chhetri DK, Berke GS. Treatment of adductor spasmodic dysphonia with selective laryngeal adductor denervation and reinnervation surgery. Otolaryngol Clin North Am 2006;39(1):106-107; with permission.)

Diagnosis

A diagnosis of EVT is clinical and made by history, examination, voice and laryngoscopic findings. The presence of periodic, oscillatory motion of the larynx, palate, and/or pharynx is considered diagnostic.[19] The presence of head or extremity tremor further supports the diagnosis. Perceptually, the voice of EVT can sound similar to SD; however, the presence of symptoms across all vocal tasks, lack of response to sensory tricks, and the presence of tremor in extralaryngeal muscles can help distinguish the two (**Table 2**).[19] As discussed previously, patients with SD may have a dystonic tremor that is distinct from the tremor of EVT in that it is irregular and task specific. In addition, EVT and SD can occur simultaneously. Laryngeal electromyography can

Table 2		
Distinguishing features of spasmodic dysphonia and essential voice tremor		
	Spasmodic Dysphonia	**Essential Voice Tremor**
Task specific	Yes	No
Consistent among all forms of vocalization (including whispering, shouting, and singing)	No	Yes
Speaking voice is spontaneous normal	No	No
Responsive to sensory tricks	Yes	No
Alcohol responsive	Yes (in some patients)	Yes (in some patients)
Tremor of extralaryngeal muscles	No	Yes
Family history	12% family history of dystonia	25%–50% family history of tremor
Resting tremor of arytenoids	No	Yes

be used in cases of diagnostic uncertainty to detect rhythmic muscle contraction at a frequency of 4 Hz to 8 Hz, which is characteristic of ET.

Treatment

Botulinum toxin injections to the larynx are considered the gold standard in the treatment of EVT.[22] Treatment of the bilateral thyroarytenoid muscles with low doses of toxin, as is performed in AdSD, is the usual treatment. In patients where a vertical tremor of the larynx also is present, bilateral injection of the strap muscles at the level of the thyroid lamina is performed at a starting dose of 2.5 U/side to 5 U/side. Injections are alternated 3 weeks to 8 weeks apart to limit risk of dysphagia.[21] Botulinum toxin injections do not eliminate tremor but rather decrease its amplitude; therefore, patients often do not have the dramatic improvement that sometimes is seen after injection in SD.[19] In addition, persistent tremor of the resonating tract, including the pharynx, palate, and tongue, will continue to cause tremulousness of the voice. Injection augmentation of the vocal folds also may be performed in EVT to combat the glottic insufficiency caused by botulinum toxin injections to the vocal folds as well as to decrease vocal effort which may exacerbate vocal tremor.[23]

Propranolol and primidone generally are believed the most effective oral agents in treating ET, although only propranolol is Food and Drug Administration approved for this purpose.[24] Propranolol has been shown to cause significant vocal improvement in some patients with EVT with minimal side effects and can be considered an adjunct or alternative treatment to botulinum toxin injections.[22] Primidone also been has shown to improve the voice in some patients with EVT, however, with a much higher rate of adverse events.[25]

PARKINSON DISEASE

PD results from cell death of dopaminergic neurons in the substantia nigra of the basal ganglia.[26] It affects approximately 1 million people in the United States. In a study of 200 successive idiopathic PD patients presenting to a movement disorders clinic, more than 70% had speech impairment when speech samples were assessed by trained raters.[27]

Diagnosis

PD is diagnosed by the presence of bradykinesia plus rest tremor and/or rigidity, plus at least 2 supportive criteria without exclusion criteria or red flags.[28] Supportive criteria include

- Clear beneficial response to dopaminergic therapy
- Presence of levodopa-induced dyskinesia
- Rest tremor of a limb
- Olfactory loss or cardiac sympathetic denervation

Parkinson-plus syndromes include PD plus autonomic or supranuclear dysfunction. Multiple system atrophy is a term for autonomic dysfunction resulting in orthostatic hypotension, sphincter dysfunction, anhidrosis, and impotence. Shy-Drager syndrome is a type of multiple system atrophy in which patients may have stridor due to failure of vocal fold abduction, which typically worsens during sleep. Patients may require a tracheostomy to maintain the airway.[29]

Speech abnormalities in PD include hypophonia, breathiness, reduced pitch, vocal decay, hypokinetic dysarthria, and monotone voice. Poor breath coordination and support as well as poor sensory feedback contribute to the decreased loudness of the voice. Patients with PD also can have voice abnormalities that are characterized by rigidity, leading to a strained voice that is similar to SD.

Acoustic analysis demonstrates increased shimmer and jitter, decreased harmonic/ noise ratio, and tremor. On flexible laryngoscopy, the vocal folds may appear thin and bowed due to muscle atrophy, with abnormal phase closure and phase asymmetry, reduced vocal fold adduction, and resting tremor, which abates during phonation.[30,31] Laryngeal EMG shows reduced thyroarytenoid muscle activity.[32] Pulmonary function testing may show abnormalities of flow-volume loops with a respiratory flutter pattern, with regular and consecutive accelerations and decelerations in flow or irregular abrupt changes in flow.[33]

Treatment

Medications, such as levodopa plus carbidopa, monoamine oxidase B inhibitors, and dopamine agonists, are used for symptom management in PD but do not modify the underlying disease process. These medications increase dopamine levels in the central nervous system. Although there are no randomized controlled trials of the effect of levodopa on voice quality, a systematic review of 33 studies and 964 patients found that administration of levodopa seemed to improve aerodynamic and/or acoustic measurements in patients with PD.[34] The systematic review was limited by poor to modest quality evidence, small numbers of patients in each study, and significant heterogeneity. In advanced PD no longer responsive to medication, subthalamic nucleus deep brain stimulation is an effective treatment of motor symptoms; however, it has been found to decrease overall speech intelligibility.[35,36]

Lee Silverman Voice Treatment (LSVT), named after a woman with PD, is considered the gold standard voice therapy in PD.[37] The goal of treatment is to "speak LOUD!"[38] and patients are taught to relearn cues for the amount of effort needed to produce normal loudness. Therapy consists of hour-long sessions 4 times a week for 4 weeks with daily homework. Patients treated with LSVT showed improved loudness of sustained phonation, rainbow passage, and conversational speech immediately post-treatment and at 2 years post-treatment.[37,39] Two Cochrane reviews recently were conducted of speech and language therapy in PD. One compared different types of speech and language therapy techniques and the other compared speech and language therapy versus placebo or no intervention in PD. Due to the small size of the studies and heterogeneity among the studies, the investigators were unable to conclude whether one form of speech and language therapy was superior to another and were unable to conclude definitively that speech and language therapy was superior to placebo.[40,41] A large-scale randomized controlled trial of LSVT versus standard speech and language therapy versus control is currently being conducted in the United Kingdom.[42]

Laryngeal surgery can benefit select patients with PD with vocal complaints. Injection laryngoplasty has been used in patients with breathiness or hypophonia and accompanying vocal fold atrophy. Small studies have shown an improvement in quality of life and increased maximum phonation time, frequency, and loudness range with collagen injection.[43,44] Medialization laryngoplasty also can be performed in patients where glottic insufficiency is believed to play a significant role in their voice disorder.[45]

SUMMARY

Movement disorders of the larynx can be diagnosed accurately when the phenomenology of each disorder is well understood, a thorough history is obtained, and the patient is carefully observed and examined. Treatment should be tailored to the specific voice disorder and to the needs of each patient.

REFERENCES

1. Fahn S, Jankovic J, Hallett M. Principles and practice of movement disorders. Philadelphia: Elsevier; 2011.
2. Mor N, Simonyan K, Blitzer A. Central voice production and pathophysiology of spasmodic dysphonia. Laryngoscope 2018;128(1):177–83.
3. Hintze JM, Ludlow CL, Bansberg SF, et al. Spasmodic dysphonia: a review. part 1: pathogenic factors. Otolaryngol Head Neck Surg 2017;157(4):551–7.
4. Blitzer A, Brin MF, Stewart CF. Botulinum toxin management of spasmodic dysphonia (laryngeal dystonia): a 12-year experience in more than 900 patients. Laryngoscope 2015;125(8):1751–7.
5. Patel AB, Bansberg SF, Adler CH, et al. The Mayo Clinic Arizona spasmodic dysphonia experience: a demographic analysis of 718 patients. Ann Otol Rhinol Laryngol 2015;124(11):859–63.
6. Chitkara A, Meyer T, Keidar A, et al. Singer's dystonia: first report of a variant of spasmodic dysphonia. Ann Otol Rhinol Laryngol 2006;115(2):89–92.
7. Hintze JM, Ludlow CL, Bansberg SF, et al. Spasmodic dysphonia: a review. part 2: characterization of pathophysiology. Otolaryngol Head Neck Surg 2017; 157(4):558–64.
8. Ludlow CL, Adler CH, Berke GS, et al. Research priorities in spasmodic dysphonia. Otolaryngol Head Neck Surg 2008;139(4):495–505.
9. Kirke DN, Frucht SJ, Simonyan K. Alcohol responsiveness in laryngeal dystonia: a survey study. J Neurol 2015;262(6):1548–56.
10. Ludlow CL, Domangue R, Sharma D, et al. Consensus-based attributes for identifying patients with spasmodic dysphonia and other voice disorders. JAMA Otolaryngol Head Neck Surg 2018;144(8):657–65.
11. Stachler RJ, Francis DO, Schwartz SR, et al. Clinical practice guideline: hoarseness (dysphonia) (update) executive summary. Otolaryngol Head Neck Surg 2018;158(3):409–26.
12. Hillel AD, Maronian NC, Waugh PF, et al. Treatment of the interarytenoid muscle with botulinum toxin for laryngeal dystonia. Ann Otol Rhinol Laryngol 2004;113(5): 341–8.
13. Tang CG, Novakovic D, Mor N, et al. Onabotulinum toxin A dosage trends over time for adductor spasmodic dysphonia: a 15-year experience. Laryngoscope 2016;126(3):678–81.
14. Rumbach AF, Blitzer A, Frucht SJ, et al. An open-label study of sodium oxybate in Spasmodic dysphonia. Laryngoscope 2017;127(6):1402–7.
15. Dewan K, Berke GS. Bilateral vocal fold medialization: a treatment for abductor spasmodic dysphonia. J Voice 2017. https://doi.org/10.1016/j.jvoice.2017.09. 027.
16. Chhetri DK, Mendelsohn AH, Blumin JH, et al. Long-term follow-up results of selective laryngeal adductor denervation-reinnervation surgery for adductor spasmodic dysphonia. Laryngoscope 2006;116(4):635–42.
17. Chhetri DK, Berke GS. Treatment of adductor spasmodic dysphonia with selective laryngeal adductor denervation and reinnervation surgery. Otolaryngol Clin North Am 2006;39(1):101–9.
18. Pitman MJ. Treatment of spasmodic dysphonia with a neuromodulating electrical implant. Laryngoscope 2014;124(11):2537–43.

19. Sulica L, Louis ED. Clinical characteristics of essential voice tremor: a study of 34 cases. Laryngoscope 2010;120(3):516–28.

20. Patel A, Frucht SJ. Isolated vocal tremor as a focal phenotype of essential tremor: a retrospective case review. J Clin Mov Disord 2015;2:4.

21. Gurey LE, Sinclair CF, Blitzer A. A new paradigm for the management of essential vocal tremor with botulinum toxin. Laryngoscope 2013;123(10):2497–501.

22. Justicz N, Hapner ER, Josephs JS, et al. Comparative effectiveness of propranolol and botulinum for the treatment of essential voice tremor. Laryngoscope 2016;126(1):113–7.

23. Estes C, Sadoughi B, Coleman R, et al. A prospective crossover trial of botulinum toxin chemodenervation versus injection augmentation for essential voice tremor. Laryngoscope 2018;128(2):437–46.

24. Zesiewicz TA, Shaw JD, Allison KG, et al. Update on treatment of essential tremor. Curr Treat Options Neurol 2013;15(4):410–23.

25. Nida A, Alston J, Schweinfurth J. Primidone therapy for essential vocal tremor. JAMA Otolaryngol Head Neck Surg 2016;142(2):117–21.

26. Damier P, Hirsch EC, Agid Y, et al. The substantia nigra of the human brain. II. Patterns of loss of dopamine-containing neurons in Parkinson's disease. Brain 1999;122(Pt 8):1437–48.

27. Ho AK, Iansek R, Marigliani C, et al. Speech impairment in a large sample of patients with Parkinson's disease. Behav Neurol 1998;11(3):131–7.

28. Postuma RB, Berg D, Stern M, et al. MDS clinical diagnostic criteria for Parkinson's disease. Mov Disord 2015;30(12):1591–601.

29. Harcourt J, Spraggs P, Mathias C, et al. Sleep-related breathing disorders in the Shy-Drager syndrome. Observations on investigation and management. Eur J Neurol 1996;3(3):186–90.

30. Perez KS, Ramig LO, Smith ME, et al. The Parkinson larynx: tremor and videostroboscopic findings. J Voice 1996;10(4):354–61.

31. Smith ME, Ramig LO, Dromey C, et al. Intensive voice treatment in Parkinson disease: laryngostroboscopic findings. J Voice 1995;9(4):453–9.

32. Baker KK, Ramig LO, Luschei ES, et al. Thyroarytenoid muscle activity associated with hypophonia in Parkinson disease and aging. Neurology 1998;51(6):1592–8.

33. Vincken WG, Gauthier SG, Dollfuss RE, et al. Involvement of upper-airway muscles in extrapyramidal disorders. A cause of airflow limitation. N Engl J Med 1984;311(7):438–42.

34. Lechien JR, Blecic S, Huet K, et al. Voice quality outcomes of idiopathic Parkinson's disease medical treatment: a systematic review. Clin Otolaryngol 2018;43(3):882–903.

35. Tsuboi T, Watanabe H, Tanaka Y, et al. Distinct phenotypes of speech and voice disorders in Parkinson's disease after subthalamic nucleus deep brain stimulation. J Neurol Neurosurg Psychiatry 2015;86(8):856–64.

36. Tripoliti E, Zrinzo L, Martinez-Torres I, et al. Effects of subthalamic stimulation on speech of consecutive patients with Parkinson disease. Neurology 2011;76(1):80–6.

37. Ramig LO, Countryman S, O'Brien C, et al. Intensive speech treatment for patients with Parkinson's disease: short-and long-term comparison of two techniques. Neurology 1996;47(6):1496–504.

38. LSVT LOUD® Treatment. LSVT LOUD® treatment 2018. Available at: https://www.lsvtglobal.com/LSVTLoud. Accessed September 6, 2018.

39. Ramig LO, Sapir S, Countryman S, et al. Intensive voice treatment (LSVT) for patients with Parkinson's disease: a 2 year follow up. J Neurol Neurosurg Psychiatry 2001;71(4):493–8.
40. Herd CP, Tomlinson CL, Deane KH, et al. Speech and language therapy versus placebo or no intervention for speech problems in Parkinson's disease. Cochrane Database Syst Rev 2012:CD002812. https://doi.org/10.1002/14651858.CD002812. pub2.
41. Herd CP, Tomlinson CL, Deane KH, et al. Comparison of speech and language therapy techniques for speech problems in Parkinson's disease. Cochrane Database Syst Rev 2012:CD002814. https://doi.org/10.1002/14651858.CD002814. pub2.
42. Sackley CM, Smith CH, Rick CE, et al. Lee Silverman Voice Treatment versus standard speech and language therapy versus control in Parkinson's disease: a pilot randomised controlled trial (PD COMM pilot). Pilot Feasibility Stud 2018; 4:30.
43. Hill AN, Jankovic J, Vuong KDAT, et al. Treatment of hypophonia with collagen vocal cord augmentation in patients with parkinsonism. Mov Disord 2003; 18(10):1190–2.
44. Sewall GK, Jiang J, Ford CN. Clinical evaluation of Parkinson's-related dysphonia. Laryngoscope 2006;116(10):1740–4.
45. Roubeau B, Bruel M, de Crouy Chanel O, et al. Reduction of Parkinson's-related dysphonia by thyroplasty. Eur Ann Otorhinolaryngol Head Neck Dis 2016;133(6): 437–9.

The Art of Caring for the Professional Singer

Adam D. Rubin, MD[a,b,c],*, Juliana Codino, MS, CCC-SLP[a,d]

KEYWORDS

- Vocal health • Laryngology • Voice pathology • Voice classification • Vocal injury
- Voice team • Singing voice • Dysphonia

KEY POINTS

- Caring for the professional singer goes beyond the basic understanding of voice evaluation, imaging, and microlaryngeal surgery.
- To treat the singer well, the otolaryngologist should be familiar with the different genres of singing, voice classification, and general singing vocabulary.
- To treat the singer well, the otolaryngologist should understand the demands of the different types of professional singers.
- The otolaryngologist should understand how to take a good voice history and recognize vocal pathology when listening to the voice.
- The otolaryngologist should not venture beyond his or her comfort level when caring for the professional singer.

INTRODUCTION

Training in care of the voice for the general otolaryngologist has improved with the presence of more fellowship-trained laryngologists within residency programs. However, preparation for caring for the professional singer goes beyond the basic understanding of laryngeal imaging and microlaryngeal surgery. There is an "art" to caring for such patients. Mastering this art will help foster trust, and lead to fruitful, rewarding relationships with the injured singer. This article is meant to introduce the otolaryngologist to the specifics of caring for professional singers. It is the responsibility of the physician to understand his or her limitations and not venture beyond, so as not to put the patient's career at risk.

No financial disclosures.
[a] Lakeshore Professional Voice Center, Lakeshore Ear, Nose & Throat Center, 21000 East 12 Mile Road Suite 111, St Clair Shores, MI 48081, USA; [b] Oakland University William Beaumont School of Medicine, Rochester, MI, USA; [c] Michigan State University College of Osteopathic Medicine, University of Michigan, MI, USA; [d] University of Buenos Aires, Buenos Aires, Argentina
* Corresponding author. Lakeshore Professional Voice Center, Lakeshore Ear, Nose & Throat Center, 21000 East 12 Mile Road Suite 111, St Clair Shores, MI 48081, USA.
E-mail address: arubin@lakeshoreent.com

0030-6665/19/© 2019 Elsevier Inc. All rights reserved.

THE VOICE TEAM

The management of the professional singer is best performed with a voice team. The team ideally would include a fellowship-trained laryngologist; a speech-language pathologist (SLP) specialized in voice disorders, ideally with a singing background; a singing voice specialist (often an SLP with experience as a voice teacher and/or performer, frequently with a bachelor's or master's degree in vocal performance); and the singing teacher. However, lack of fellowship training should not preclude the general otolaryngologist or speech pathologist in caring for such patients if they have the interest. As many general otolaryngologists will not have a speech pathologist working in the same office, it is important to identify one in the community with training and experience in voice. Communication among all team members is critical to formulate an integrated and practical treatment plan. Inclusion of the singing teacher is important to receive his or her perspective, share your findings, and to not make the teacher feel alienated or insulted. However, the team must also assess whether the singing teacher is providing appropriate training for the patient. Monitoring of progress may include follow-up videostroboscopies; perceptual, acoustical, and aerodynamic data; as well as self-assessment tools. A key ingredient is the performer's openness and commitment to retrain or rehabilitate his or her voice.

THE INITIAL VISIT

The initial encounter with the patient is critical for making a connection with the patient and establishing trust. A good singing voice history is important to not only find out exactly what bothers the patient, but also to listen to the quality of the voice and observe how the patient is speaking. Singers are particularly "in-tune" with their voices. They may explain that their range is affected, their voice is fatiguing more easily, there is a break in the *passagio* that was not there previously, or maybe things just do not "feel right." To take a good history, the physician must have basic knowledge of the different genres of music, voice types, and vocabulary of the profession to win the confidence of the patient.

GENRES OF MUSIC

There are numerous different genres of singing, all of which offer different challenges and advantages for vocal health. For example, popular singing allows for the use of amplification, which when used appropriately can alleviate vocal strain even in extremes of range. Some of the more well-known genres include classical, jazz, musical theater, gospel, blues, country, pop, and rock. But there are numerous others with various cultural backgrounds: African, Indian, East Asian, and Caribbean, for example, Some of these create sounds that are formed with more tension and can create challenges for the patient and the treatment. Moreover, within each genre, there are numerous different styles. For example, in musical theater there are roles that require more "legit" or lyrical singing and those that require a "belt." Belting describes a powerful sound, with penetrating intensity that may imitate speechlike inflections in a higher than usual range for the singer's speaking voice. Singers belt when they sing in their modal register ("chest voice") certain tones that actually belong to their "head voice" or higher register. Belting done incorrectly can put a voice at great risk for injury. It is wise for the clinician to be familiar with the different musical genres and styles of singing, as well as names of composers and leading performers within each genre.

CLASSICAL SINGING

Classically trained singers will often have had the most sophisticated training and repertoire. The otolaryngologist must approach this subject delicately and explain that therapy is geared to treat the injured voice, not to teach them how to sing. One might explain that even with great technique, a voice can be injured. Also, although most singers have excellent training in the singing voice, few have training in the speaking voice.

The classical singer is usually staged without electronic amplification and must perform in various acoustical settings. Their primary means of portraying a character is with the voice. Usually, the vocal challenges involve a wide pitch and amplitude range, specific timbre that the musical director or composer dictates, and long duration of phrases. Moreover, they must embody the emotions of the character while being heard over an orchestra and/or choir. One of the tools the classically trained singer uses do this is the singer's formant.[1]

VOICE CLASSIFICATION

Voice classification is based on several qualities of the singing voice and helps singers choose appropriate repertoire and roles. Such parameters include the following:

- Vocal range
- *Passagio*
- *Tessitura*

Vocal range is the span of pitches the voice can produce. Some singers will know their exact range and describe it by keys on a piano. C1 is the lowest C on the piano keyboard, whereas C4 is middle C. The *tessitura* is the range of frequencies that a singer can produce in a comfortable, easy way. The extension, however, is the total range of musical tones that a singer can vocalize with effort. This latter represents the laryngeal capacity, but is not as crucial for voice classification purposes.

Certain anatomic features are common among specific voice types (vocal fold thickness, length of vocal tract), which may contribute to voice classification. Acoustical parameters, such as timbre, intensity, vocal agility, and vibrato, will contribute to voice classification, but their main use is for voice subclassification. Timbre refers to the color or tone of the sound. The timbre will sound best in a singer's *tessitura*. Vibrato is a musical effect produced by regular rapid change in pitch during sustained phonation. It can be characterized by its extent (range of pitch variation) and rate (speed of its variation).

The basic voice classification involves the following voice types:

- For female singers:
  - Soprano
  - Mezzo-soprano
  - Alto
- For male singers:
  - Counter-tenor
  - Tenor
  - Baritone
  - Bass

Each of these is listed from highest pitch range to lowest. There are also subclassifications within each voice type (**Table 1**). Some singers might describe themselves with some variation. For example, a baritone with a lighter quality to the voice and high extension, might call himself a "bari-tenor."

Table 1		
Voice classification and subclassification with the corresponding *tessitura*		
Voice Classification	*Tessitura*	Subclassification
Soprano	C4-C6	*Leggera, coloratura,* lyric, dramatic, *spinto*
Mezzo-soprano	A3-A5	*Leggera,* lyric, dramatic
Alto	F3-F5	Lyric, dramatic, *buffa*
Tenor	C3-C5	*Leggero,* lyric, dramatic, *spinto, buffo*
Baritone	A2-A4	*Leggero,* lyric, dramatic, *buffo*
Bass	E2-E4	Lyric, *buffo, profondo*

REGISTER AND *PASSAGIO*

The term register has been described perceptually as "distinct regions of vocal quality that can be maintained over some ranges of pitch and loudness."[2] Simply put, from low to high, the registers are as follows:

- Glottal fry (pulse)
- Modal (chest)
- Head voice (falsetto)
- Whistle (in women)

On an ascending *glissando* (sliding from a low note to a high note), these changes in register can be heard and are visible within acoustical data (spectrogram, oscillogram, electroglottogram) as disruptions in the signal related to an upward jump in fundamental frequency. The complexity of vocal registers is beyond the scope of this article. A recent theory explains the phenomenon through the mutually antagonistic functions of shortening and thickening the thyroarytenoid and the lengthening and thinning of the cricothyroid muscles.[3]

Smoothing the transition between laryngeal registers is one of the challenges of singing technique. The transition between registers is called the *passagio*. The *passagio* is a sensitive area for vibratory impairment. A new break in the *passagio* in a well-trained singer usually signifies some source of vibratory impairment, whereas it is common to hear a disruption in the sound in an untrained voice.

DYNAMICS

Dynamics refers to loudness of a phrase or section of a musical piece. *Piano* (*p*) indicates soft, and *forte* (*f*), indicates loud. There are variations, such as *mezzo-piano* (*mp*) or *mezzo-forte* (*mf*), indicating "medium" soft or loud. Others include *pianissimo* (*pp*) and *fortissimo* (*ff*), meaning very soft and very loud. It is important to explore the patient's range at different dynamic levels.

NONCLASSICAL SINGING

Nonclassical singing includes almost every other genre. The vocal demands or requirements in many popular styles are different compared with classical singing. Popular singing styles usually use amplification; a jazz singer, for example, should have a decent amplification system that will help his or her voice to be heard over the band. So these types of music styles do not need as much vocal tract adjustments as the classical singer who usually is using his or her resonance system to stand out above the orchestra and choir. This goes hand in hand with articulatory agility: many popular singing styles prioritize lyrics intelligibility, so because they do not need significant adaptations in their vocal tracts for amplification purposes allows them to have good intelligibility. In contrast, the classical singer will focus on timbre, volume, and desired sound at times at the expense of understandability. Some popular styles are performed while dancing or doing specific body movements that jeopardize healthy vocal production. The voice team needs to observe how this is performed and make sure the patient is doing it in a way that avoids vocal injury.

HISTORY

Much of the basic history taken from a professional singer is similar to that taken from any voice patient. For example, acuity of onset and preceding event will investigate whether the incident is due to a phonotraumatic event. Progression versus intermittency suggests different potential etiologies. An excellent question to ask is if the voice returns to normal with rest. If so, this would argue against a major structural abnormality, and perhaps the problem is more related to overuse or other factors. Exploring environmental factors and phonotraumatic habits will yield useful information.

Questions that will help the singer formulate his or her history include "What is your voice doing that it should not do?" or "What is your voice not doing that it should do?" Asking the singer what the general concerns are will allow him or her to try to articulate the problem. However, the physician can assist, while demonstrating an understanding of the profession, by asking questions concerning how the range is affected or what part of the register is problematic. As mentioned, the *passagio* is a particularly sensitive area to vibratory impairment. Asking about the ability to sing softly in the upper range is important, as belting or loud singing will allow for subtle vibratory abnormalities to be unnoticed due to the compensatory effect of added support and volume.

It is important to get a sense of the level of difficulty of the music being performed. Is it in the patient's *tessitura*? Some nonclassical singers might not be familiar with this term, so one should ask if it rests in a comfortable range. One common problem in choir singing is stronger singers being asked to sing a different voice part to strengthen that section. A contralto might be asked to sing soprano, for example. She may be able to hit the higher notes, but they might not be in her *tessitura*.

It is important to assess how well-trained the singer is. Many rock, jazz, or blues singers go by "God-given talent," whereas many well-trained singers have had no speaking training. This becomes particularly relevant in the musical theater performer who has significant speaking parts, particularly if these parts tend to be dramatic or emotional. In addition to inquiring about how many years of training the singer has, it is important to know if it was continuous or interrupted. Inquiring how many teachers he or she has studied with and how long he or she has been with the last is important. If someone has trained for 20 years, but has had 5 different teachers, he or she might not have solid technique.

Performance environment can have an effect on one's vocal health. Older theaters might have issues with dust or mildew. Use of fog machines and pyrotechnics have been shown to affect the voice.[4,5] Rock singers might be performing in smoky bars. It is important to inquire about equipment use, particularly the use of monitors. In general, one wants to assess if acoustics are being optimized and environmental irritants minimized. The traveling performer can be particularly challenged. Sleep deprivation, poor diet, and a multitude of different venues can create significant stress on the voice.

Assessing the vocal demands placed on the patient is vital. How many performances are there a week? How many practices? Are they being asked to sing full out during rehearsals, or are they permitted to mark? What other demands are on them not related to their performance schedule? Are they waiting tables or have some other vocally demanding day-job? Are they going home and resting after performances, or going to a bar to have a few drinks and a late-night meal? Exploring all aspects of vocal hygiene is obviously important.

Asking about general health issues, such as allergies and reflux, is necessary, as well as review of the patient's medications. One should look for medications that could be drying systemically or causing direct irritation to the vocal folds. Anticholinergics and inhalers tend to be common culprits.

Last, but not least, the physician should get a sense of the performer's mental and emotional state. Voice problems in professional singers create a great deal of anxiety. One needs to explore what the singer is afraid of most. One has to explore the short-term and long-term goals of the professional and assess what is most important to the patient at that moment in time. Furthermore, some performers experience stage fright despite being experienced and well-trained. This can affect the patient's technique and vocal health (**Table 2**).

TO PULL OR NOT TO PULL THE PERFORMER OFF STAGE

One of the most important decisions that the voice team will need to make is whether to pull a performer off stage. The decision should not be taken lightly, as it could have significant repercussions, not only in the short-run, but also for the patient's career. The patient is faced with the dilemma of risking further injury, performing badly, or developing a reputation of being unreliable. All of these factors could make the difference in determining future success.

Furthermore, although the number 1 responsibility is to the patient's well-being, the patient and physician have to consider the ramifications of the decision. Is there an understudy? How large is the role? Will the tour or production be canceled? What are the financial consequences? Will the rock-and-roll singer miss an opportunity for large financial windfall by canceling the tour? Depending on the patient's wishes, one might want to involve the director and/or producer in the discussion.

That said, the number one concern for the physician should be the safety of the patient. One wants to avoid a potentially career-ending vocal injury - deep vocal fold scar. Two indications for absolute voice rest include vocal fold hemorrhage and tear. A deep hemorrhage may require 6 weeks off singing, whereas a tear typically will heal with a few days of voice rest. Other reasons for relative voice rest include a phonotraumatic or viral laryngitis. In these cases, discussion and potential for medical management will guide the team to the best decision.[6]

Other things to investigate include the following:

1. Does the patient have a major role, or just a cameo?
2. What type of music is it?
3. Can he or she perform the role adequately?
4. Can the patient be helped with additional amplification or effects?
5. Is there a way to modify the performance?

Performance modification can include suggestions such as changing the melodies (not possible in theater or opera, but possible for a cover band), revising the repertoire,

Table 2
Risk factors and vocal hygiene in singers

Voice and repertoire	• Inadequate training • Repertoire is outside of the singer's *tessitura* • Range is too challenging • Singing outside appropriate voice type in choir to fill in need of weaker section • Going out after performances, not allowing for voice recovery • Poor vocal hygiene
Economic factors	• Having a vocally demanding "day-job" • Booking more obligations than voice can withstand • Meet and greet after concerts • Needing to perform when vocally compromised
Posture	• Playing an instrument simultaneously onstage • Stages with incline affecting singer's body alignment • Choreographer's or director's demands for challenging postures, movements, or dancing while singing
Performer's psyche and general health	• Stage fright and vocal *trac* (from French word *tracasser*, to bother or to worry) • Fear of introducing voice technique modifications even when they will be effective • Stress • Emotional weakness or instability • "Pushing," feeling the need to give "200%" • Excessive travel: sleep deprivation, poor diet • Medications that irritate or dry • Allergies • Reflux • Other medical problems
Costumes and props	• Uncomfortable costumes that impair comfortable movement • Exceptionally fast costume changes • Artificial beards or mustaches, masks that limit articulatory ability or vocal perception • Heavy wigs or hats that cause cervical spine tension • Uncomfortable shoes affecting posture and balance • Makeup, hairspray that might be irritating
Rehearsals	• Rehearsal space is different from performance space • Demanding "tech week" • Too many rehearsals or rehearsals that are too long can be fatiguing even with good technique • Music directors not allowing marking • Poor marking technique • Wanting to sound at performance quality during rehearsal to impress colleagues
Environment	• Environmental irritants (fog machines,[6] dust, smoke) • Excessive background noise • Poor acoustics • Lack of monitors

saving on group numbers or backup singing, and marking rehearsals. This last suggestion is particularly important. One should remind the patient that he or she does not need to show everyone his or her talent at rehearsal. The patient should save it for the performance. Of course, the performer must know how to appropriately mark as singing more softly can sometime erroneously be done with more tension. Taking melodies an octave down can also be voice-preserving in the rehearsal setting. Staging and choreography do not require all-out singing to be designed and rehearsed.[6]

One particularly important element to discern in the history is how much the patient is "pushing" during rehearsals and performances. Singers and actors feel the performance will be that much better with more "energy." They tend to want to give "200%." In truth, the secret to a long and healthy acting and performing career is to find out how little energy needs to be exerted for an effective performance. At a point, additional effort might not only be harmful, but can actually make the performance less believable. In stage-acting, pushing too much can "break the fourth wall" and make the performance less believable.[6]

MEDICAL TREATMENT OF THE PERFORMER

The challenges of performance careers today are great. The otolaryngologist and speech pathologist must be active participants to help keep performers on stage, while minimizing the risk for injury. This, unfortunately, can lead to potential overuse of medications, such as glucocorticoids, which can have tremendously beneficial effects on the voice when there is inflammation from overuse or illness. However, the physician must balance the beneficial effects with the potential short-term and long-term sequelae of this medication.

Other medications can be useful for particular maladies, including allergies, reflux, upper respiratory infections, and other systemic disorders. Discussion of management of these issues is beyond the scope of this article. In addition, the physician should explore what homeopathic remedies the patient is using. Some of these can be detrimental to the patient's health over the long term.

PHYSICAL EXAMINATION

The details of the examination of the injured singer is beyond the scope of the article; however, it is important to listen to the quality of the voice to have an idea what one might find on examination. If one knows what one is looking for, one is more likely to find it, rather than attribute persistent dysphonia to reflux or allergy. For example, if there is roughness or raspiness to the voice, this signifies impairment in vibration. Breathiness to the voice signifies impairment in closure, and a change in resonance would indicate a problem in the supraglottic tract. Loss of range could be due to a mass, increased stiffness to the vocal fold, or impairment in superior laryngeal nerve function.[6]

Videostroboscopy is imperative to evaluate the vibratory characteristics of the vocal fold. If one suspects an impairment in vibration, one might wish to start with rigid videostroboscopy, which provides more magnification than a flexible examination. Although, if one predominantly appreciates breathiness or altered resonance, starting with a flexible examination would be appropriate. However, if one does not see pathology to explain what one hears in the voice, one must evaluate the adequacy of the examination.

VOICE THERAPY

Voice rehabilitation in performers should address the injured mechanism reassuring the patient that the clinician will be working from a physiologic standpoint. The voice therapist or singing voice specialist may transition the patient to singing voice, however, one should communicate with the patient's singing teacher during this transition. He or she will aim to add resources to rehabilitate the injury and to maintain a healthy vocal mechanism.

In the case of acute vocal injuries, apart from the different levels of voice rest, vocal fold tissue mobilization in the form of specific voice therapy exercises (mostly voiceless or low-impact vocal fold vibrations) have been shown to limit the influx of inflammatory mediators into the tissue while increasing concentrations of anti-inflammatory mediators released by tissue motion.[7]

SURGERY

The principles of microlaryngeal surgery are the same for the singer as they are for phonotraumatic lesions in other professions; however, there is less room for error. This surgery should be performed only if the surgeon is comfortable with his or her experience and skill set, and has the appropriate equipment to treat the patient. Furthermore, one must be certain that the mass is the cause of the presenting dysphonia. Many performers sing well despite small masses on the vocal folds. However, they may present because a separate issue is creating problems. Moreover, sometimes masses will give the performer a certain character to the voice that distinguishes him or her and is part of the reason for his or her success. Removal of such a mass could jeopardize a patient's career. This quagmire often arises in evaluating the traveling performer. Often the otolaryngologist is meeting the patient for the first time without any prior knowledge of the patient's voice or anatomy. Singers are encouraged to get a baseline stroboscopy when healthy. It is easy for them to store their videos on a cell phone so it is with them to access at any time. Ultimately, an otolaryngologist should venture to surgical intervention only when he or she is certain a mass is the issue, will not or has not responded to therapy, and feels comfortable with microlaryngeal surgery.

SUMMARY

Treatment of the singer can be both challenging and rewarding. The otolaryngologist should be familiar with the demands of different musical genres and obligations. He or she should be familiar with the vocabulary of singing to understand the patient's issues as well as to establish trust with the singer. Establishment of a voice team, acquiring and mastering the equipment necessary to evaluate and treat high-end singers, and devoting the time to learn more about the field, will prepare the otolaryngologist to care for this population. The otolaryngologist should only venture as far as he or she feels comfortable, as the margin for error in the treatment of the singer is small.

REFERENCES

1. Sundberg J. Articulatory interpretation of the "singing formant." J Acoust Soc Am 1974;55:838.
2. Titze IR. A framework for the study of vocal registers. J Voice 1988;2:183–94.
3. Pinho S, Pontes P. Musculos intrinsecos da laringe e dinamica vocal. Serie Desvendando os segredos da voz, vol. 1. Rio de Janeiro, Brazil: Livaria e Editor Revinter Ltda; 2008.
4. Rossol M. Artificial fogs and smokes. In: Sataloff RT, editor. Professional voice: the science and art of clinical care. 4th edition. San Diego (CA): Plural Publishing; 2017.

5. Del'Aria C, Opperman DA. Pyrotechnics in the entertainment industry: an overview. In: Sataloff RT, editor. Professional voice: the science and art of clinical care. 4th edition. San Diego (CA): Plural Publishing; 2017.
6. Rubin A. The vocal pitstop. Devon, UK: Compton Publishing; 2014.
7. Verdolini Abbott K, Li N, Branski R, et al. Vocal exercise may attenuate acute vocal fold inflammation. J Voice 2012;26(6):814.

Moving?

Make sure your subscription moves with you!

To notify us of your new address, find your **Clinics Account Number** (located on your mailing label above your name), and contact customer service at:

Email: journalscustomerservice-usa@elsevier.com

800-654-2452 (subscribers in the U.S. & Canada)
314-447-8871 (subscribers outside of the U.S. & Canada)

Fax number: 314-447-8029

Elsevier Health Sciences Division
Subscription Customer Service
3251 Riverport Lane
Maryland Heights, MO 63043

*To ensure uninterrupted delivery of your subscription, please notify us at least 4 weeks in advance of move.

Printed and bound by CPI Group (UK) Ltd, Croydon, CR0 4YY

03/10/2024

01040481-0017